Department of the Army's First Aid Manual

TC 4-02.1

Headquarters, Department of the Army

JANUARY 2016

Made available by:

Prepper Press

Post-Apocalyptic Fiction & Survival Nonfiction

www.PrepperPress.com

ISBN: 978-1-939473-84-4

Printed in the United States of America

Cover Photo: U.S. Soldiers assigned to Charlie Company, 173rd Airborne Brigade perform first aid on a mannequin during training exercise Saber Junction 2014 at the Joint Multinational Readiness Center in Hohenfels, Germany, Aug. 27, 2014. Saber Junction 2014 prepares U.S., NATO allies and European security partners to conduct unified land operations through the simultaneous combination of offensive, defensive and stability operations appropriate to the mission and the environment.

U.S. Army photo by Spc. Brian Chaney/Released

Change 1
Training Circular
No. 4-02.1

Headquarters
Department of the Army
Washington, DC, 5 August 2016

FIRST AID

1. Change Training Circular (TC) 4-02.1, dated 21 January 2016, as follows:

Remove Old Pages	Insert New Pages
iii through vi	iii through vi
pages 1-7 through 1-8	pages 1-7 through 1-8
N/A	pages 24-1 through 27-2
References-1 and References-2	References-1 and References-2

2. New or changed material is indicated by a star (★).

3. File this transmittal sheet in front of the publication.

By Order of the Secretary of the Army:

MARK A. MILLEY
General, United States Army
Chief of Staff

GERALD B. O'KEEFE
Administrative Assistant to the
Secretary of the Army
1621802

Training Circular (TC)
No. 4-02.1

Headquarters
Department of the Army
Washington, DC, 21 January 2016

First Aid

Contents

***This publication supersedes FM 4-25.11/NTRP 4-02.1.1/AFMAN 44-163(I)/MCRP 3-02G, dated 23 December 2002.**

Figures

Preface

Training Circular (TC) 4-02.1 provides first aid techniques and guidance for Soldiers. Implementation of the techniques presented in this publication enable Soldiers to render first aid and prevent greater harm to injured Soldiers.

The principal audience for TC 4-02.1 is commanders, subordinate leaders, individual Soldiers, Department of Defense (DOD) civilians and contractors.

Commanders, staffs, and subordinates ensure their decisions and actions comply with applicable United States, international, and, in some cases, host-nation laws and regulations. Commanders at all levels ensure their Soldiers operate in accordance with the law of war and the rules of engagement. (Refer to Field Manual [FM] 27-10.)

This publication is in consonance with the following North Atlantic Treaty Organization (NATO) Standards and Standardization Agreements (STANAGs):

Title	STANAGs	Standards
Allied Medical Publication (AMedP), Military Acute Trauma Care Training		8.12
Requirement for Training in First-Aid, Emergency Care in Combat Situations and Basic Hygiene for all Military Personnel	2122	
First-Aid Dressings, First Aid Kits and Emergency Medical Care Kits	2126	
First Aid and Hygiene Training in a Chemical, Biological, Radiological, and Nuclear or Toxic Industrial Hazard Environment	2358	
Requirements for Military Acute Trauma Care Training	2544	

This publication uses joint terms where applicable. Selected joint and Army terms and definitions appear in both the glossary and the text. This publication is not the proponent for any Army terms. Unless otherwise stated in this publication, the use of masculine nouns and pronouns does not refer exclusively to men.

Training Circular 4-02.1 applies to the Active Army, Army National Guard/Army National Guard of the United States, and United States Army Reserve unless otherwise stated.

The proponent and the preparing agency of this publication is the United States Army Medical Department Center and School, United States Army Health Readiness Center of Excellence. Send comments and recommendations on a DA Form 2028 (Recommended Changes to Publications and Blank Forms) to **Commander, United States Army Medical Department Center and School, United States Army Health Readiness Center of Excellence, ATTN: MCCS-FDL (TC 4-02.1), 2377 Greeley Road, Building 4011, Suite D, JBSA Fort Sam Houston, Texas 78234-7731**; by e-mail to usarmy.jbsa.medcom-ameddcs.mbx.ameddcs-medical-doctrine@mail.mil; or submit an electronic DA Form 2028. Recommended changes should be keyed to the specific page, paragraph, and line number. A rationale for each proposed change is required to aid in the evaluation and adjudication of each comment.

Introduction

Because medical personnel will not always be readily available, nonmedical Soldiers must rely on themselves and other Soldiers' skills and knowledge of first aid methods to render aid until medical assistance arrives. First aid is given until medical care provided by medically trained personnel such as a combat medic or other health care provider arrives.

The individual being provided first aid (by self-aid, buddy aid, or combat lifesaver) is considered a casualty. Once medically trained personnel (combat medic, paramedic, or other health care provider) initiates care, the casualty is then considered to be a patient.

Training Circular 4-02.1 provides first aid procedures for nonmedical personnel in environments from home station to combat situations. This publication is meant to be used by trainers and individuals being trained based on common first aid tasks. Tasks are found in the Soldier's Manual of Common Tasks, Warrior Skills Level 1, and appropriate modified tasks from the Soldier's Manual and Trainer's Guide, Military Occupational Specialty (MOS) 68W. These tasks are meant to reinforce and maintain proficiency in correct procedures for giving first aid throughout a Soldier's time in Service.

Training Circular 4-02.1 is designed to facilitate training and first aid competencies by bridging first aid training across the spectrum of assignments from training to permanent duty station and deployment. Tactical combat casualty care (TC3) is introduced in TC 4-02.1 with first aid tasks and procedures associated with combat situations. Individual and multiple first aid tasks in combination with collective tasks, may be integrated into various training scenarios.

★ This is a complete revision of FM 4-25.11/NTRP 4-02.1/AFMAN 44-163(I)/MCRP 3-02G that transforms the publication to an Army training circular. It is designed to facilitate training individual tasks and combining those tasks into logical and progressive training opportunities from individual, small unit, subsequently integrated into larger and more complex training scenarios. The purpose is to integrate and maintain first aid proficiency throughout the depth and breadth of the Army formation.

★ There are 27 chapters each covering an individual first aid task and one appendix describing and listing the contents of the United States Army Improved First Aid Kit (IFAK) and the new IFAK II.

This revision and transformation of the first aid publication supports the United States Army Doctrine 2015 initiative.

Chapter 1
Fundamentals of First Aid

1-1. When a nonmedical Soldier encounters an unconscious or injured Soldier, he must quickly and accurately evaluate the situation and the casualty to determine if it is safe for him to act as well as what, if any, first aid measures may be needed to prevent further injury or death. He should ask if trained medical personnel are available or direct someone else at the scene to call for or locate trained medical personnel. To prevent further injury to the casualty, once first aid has begun to be administered there should be no interruptions and those efforts should continue until such time as that Soldier is relieved by medical personnel. Soldiers may also have to depend upon their own first aid knowledge and skills to save themselves (self-aid). A thorough understanding of the fundamentals of first aid can save a life, prevent permanent disability, or reduce long periods of hospitalization by knowing WHAT to do, WHAT NOT to do, and WHEN to do it.

SECTION I — TERMINOLOGY

1-2. The following key terms are identified and described in order to provide a further understanding of first aid. The key terms are presented in alphabetical order, not in order of importance.

KEY TERMS

1-3. Knowledge of a few key terms will help Soldiers to better understand and appreciate the role that they play when providing first aid in tactical and nontactical environments. These terms include—

- Casualty evacuation (CASEVAC).
- Combat lifesaver.
- Combat medic.
- Emergency medical treatment.
- Enhanced first aid.
- First aid (self-aid and buddy aid).
- Medical evacuation.
- Medical treatment.
- Medical treatment facility.
- Tactical combat casualty care.

DEFINITIONS OF KEY TERMS

1-4. Knowing the key terms as they are used in Army doctrine assists in the understanding of when and how Soldiers provide first aid procedures in garrison or when deployed.

Casualty Evacuation

1-5. Nonmedical units use this to refer to the movement of casualties aboard nonmedical vehicles or aircraft without en route medical care.

Combat Lifesaver

1-6. Combat lifesavers are nonmedical Soldiers selected by their unit commander for additional training beyond basic first aid procedures. Combat lifesavers provide enhanced first aid for injuries.

Combat Medic

1-7. Combat medics are the first individuals in the medical chain that make medically substantiated decisions based on medical MOS-specific training.

Emergency Medical Treatment

1-8. Emergency medical treatment is the immediate application of medical procedures to the wounded, injured, or sick by specially trained medical personnel.

Enhanced First Aid

1-9. Enhanced first aid is administered by the combat lifesaver. It includes measures, which require an additional level of training above self-aid and buddy aid.

First Aid (Self-Aid and Buddy Aid)

1-10. Urgent and immediate lifesaving and other measures which can be performed for casualties (or performed by the casualty himself) by nonmedical personnel when medical personnel are not immediately available.

Medical Evacuation

1-11. Medical evacuation is the process of moving any person who is wounded, injured, or ill to and/or between medical treatment facilities while providing en route medical care. Also referred to as *MEDEVAC* in relation to the 9-line medical evacuation request.

Medical Treatment

1-12. Medical treatment is the care and management of wounded, injured, or ill personnel by medically trained personnel.

Medical Treatment Facility

1-13. Medical treatment facility is any facility established for the purpose of providing medical treatment. This includes battalion aid stations, Role 2 facilities, dispensaries, clinics, and hospitals.

Tactical Combat Casualty Care

1-14. Tactical combat casualty care is often referred to as TC3. Tactical combat casualty care is prehospital care provided in a tactical-combat setting. Tactical combat casualty care is divided into the following three stages:

- Care under fire.
- Tactical field care.
- Tactical evacuation.

SECTION II — VITAL BODY SYSTEMS

1-15. Basic understanding of vital body systems is crucial in the understanding and performance of first aid. Understanding vital body systems not only assists in first aid, but prevents doing any more harm to the casualty.

UNDERSTANDING VITAL BODY SYSTEMS

1-16. For Soldiers to perform first aid effectively they must have a basic understanding of the structure and function of these vital body systems. These systems are the respiratory system, the circulatory system, and the musculoskeletal system. Injury to or compromise of these systems can quickly result in permanent injury or death of the injured.

RESPIRATORY SYSTEM

1-17. Human beings require oxygen to live. Through the breathing process (respiration), the lungs draw oxygen from the air and transfer it to the red blood cells within the circulatory system.

1-18. The normal range of respirations varies based on the age and physical condition of the individual at rest. For example—

- Adults 12 to 20 breaths per minute.
- Children (1 to 10 years): 15 to 30 breaths per minute.
- Infants (6 to 12 months): 25 to 50 breaths per minute.
- Infants (0 to 5 months): 25 to 40 breaths per minute.

COMPONENTS OF THE RESPIRATORY SYSTEM

1-19. The respiratory system consists of the—

- Airway.
- Lungs.
- Rib cage.

AIRWAY

1-20. The airway consists of the nose, mouth, throat, voice box, and windpipe. It is the canal through which air passes to and from the lungs.

LUNGS

1-21. The lungs are two elastic organs made up of thousands of tiny air sacs and covered by an airtight membrane.

RIB CAGE

1-22. The rib cage is formed by the muscle-connected ribs, which join the spine in back and the breastbone in front.

CIRCULATORY SYSTEM

1-23. The circulatory system provides the vehicle for oxygen acquired through the respiratory process to be transported throughout the body.

COMPONENTS OF THE CIRCULATORY SYSTEM

1-24. The circulatory system consists of the—

- Heart.
- Blood.
- Blood vessels (arteries, capillaries, and veins).

THE HEART

1-25. Simply stated the heart is the engine that drives the human body. The only function of the heart is to pump blood. The right side of the heart pumps blood to the lungs, where oxygen is added to the blood and carbon dioxide is removed from it. The left side pumps blood to the rest of the body, where oxygen and nutrients are delivered to tissues and waste products (such as carbon dioxide) are transferred to the blood for removal by other organs such as the lungs and kidneys.

Heartbeat

1-26. The normal heart rate (heartbeats per minute) varies based on the age and physical condition of the individual at rest. For example—

- Adults 60 to 100 heartbeats per minute.
- Children (1 to 6 years): 70 to 120 heartbeats per minute.
- Infants (6 to 12 months): 80 to 140 heartbeats per minute.
- Infants (0 to 5 months): 90 to 140 heartbeats per minute.

Note. The typical pulse for Soldiers and athletes (40 to 60 beats per minute) is lower than the average adult population.

1-27. The heartbeat is a rhythmic cycle of contraction and relaxation of the heart muscle which causes expansion and contraction of the arteries as it forces blood through them. This cycle of expansion and contraction can be felt (monitored) at various points in the body and is called the pulse.

Pulse

1-28. The pulse is the first major indicator of the general physiological state of a casualty when Soldiers are performing a casualty assessment. The presence or absence will determine what needs to be done and the order in which those actions must be taken to preserve the life of the injured.

1-29. The points where a pulse can be readily felt are located at the following arterial points of the body:

- Carotid.
- Femoral.
- Radial.
- Posterior tibial.

Carotid Pulse

1-30. To check the carotid pulse (carotid arteries, felt at the neck), feel for a pulse on the side of the casualty's neck closest to you. This is done by placing the tips of your first two fingers beside his Adam's apple.

Femoral Pulse

1-31. To check the femoral pulse (large femoral artery located in the thigh [felt in the groin]), press the tips of your first two fingers into the middle of the groin.

Radial Pulse

1-32. To check the radial pulse (at the wrist), place your first two fingers on the thumb side of the casualty's wrist.

Posterior Tibial Pulse

1-33. To check the posterior tibial pulse (inside the big toe side of the ankle), place your first two fingers on the inside of the ankle.

Note. Do not use your thumb to check a casualty's pulse. The individual's pulse can be felt in the thumb and may confuse the beat of his pulse with that of the casualty's.

WARNING

It is imperative that first aid providers quickly determine if the casualty has a pulse (heartbeat). Absence of a pulse (heartbeat) will lead to the death of the casualty if not quickly restored.

BLOOD

1-34. If the heart is the engine that drives the body, blood is the fuel which powers and sustains the human body. Blood is a mixture of plasma (liquid component), white blood cells, red blood cells, and platelets. The body contains about 5 to 6 quarts (about 5 liters) of blood. Once blood is pumped out of the heart, it takes 20 to 30 seconds to circulate through the body and return to the heart.

1-35. Blood performs essential functions as it circulates through the body. It delivers oxygen and essential nutrients (such as fats, sugars, minerals, and vitamins) to the body's tissues. It carries carbon dioxide to the lungs and other waste products to the kidneys for elimination from the body. Also, it carries components that fight infection and stop bleeding.

WARNING

It is imperative that first aid providers quickly determine if the casualty is losing blood. Excessive loss of blood can quickly lead to the death of the casualty if not stopped.

BLOOD VESSELS

1-36. Blood vessels are the conduit which transports blood pumped by the heart to the body. The blood vessels consist of—

- Arteries.
- Arterioles.
- Capillaries.
- Venules.
- Veins.

ARTERIES

1-37. Arteries are vessels that carry blood high in oxygen content away from the heart to the farthest reaches of the body. Arteries flow into arterioles.

ARTERIOLES

1-38. Arterioles are small branches of arteries that lead to the capillaries.

CAPILLARIES

1-39. Capillaries are tiny blood vessels that connect arterioles (the smallest division of an artery) with venules.

VENULES

1-40. Venules are small veins that go from capillaries to veins.

Veins

1-41. A blood vessel that carries blood that is low in oxygen content from the body back to the heart.

> **WARNING**
>
> **It is imperative that first aid providers quickly determine if a casualty is losing blood. Many injuries can result in blood vessels being torn which result in excessive blood loss. Excessive loss of blood can quickly lead to the death of the casualty if not stopped.**

MUSCULOSKELETAL SYSTEM

1-42. The skeleton provides a structural framework for the body and, because bones are rigid, provides support and protection for vital organs and softer tissues. Skeletal muscles and bones work together to make body movement possible.

Components of the Musculoskeletal System

1-43. The musculoskeletal system is composed of—

- Bones.
- Joints.
- Muscles.
- Cartilage.
- Ligaments.
- Tendons.

Bones

1-44. Bone is the substance that forms the skeleton of the body. It is composed chiefly of calcium phosphate and calcium carbonate. The human body has 206 bones. There are 80 axial (head and trunk) bones and 126 appendicular (upper and lower extremity) bones. Bones provide structural support for the body. Individual and groups of bones provide structure for the attachment of soft tissues and protect organs.

Joints

1-45. Joints are the areas where two bones are attached for the purpose of permitting body parts to move.

Muscles

1-46. Muscle is the tissue of the body which primarily functions as a source of power. There are three types of muscle in the body. Muscle which is responsible for moving extremities and external areas of the body is called *skeletal muscle*. Heart muscle is called *cardiac muscle*. Muscle that is in the walls of arteries and bowel is called *smooth muscle*.

Cartilage

1-47. Cartilage is a firm, rubbery tissue that cushions bones at joints. A flexible kind of cartilage makes up other parts of the body, such as the larynx and the outside parts of the ears.

LIGAMENTS

1-48. Ligaments are a tough band of connective tissue that connects various structures, such as two bones.

TENDONS

1-49. Tendons are a soft tissue by which muscle attaches to bone. Tendons are somewhat flexible, but tough.

SECTION III — GENERAL PRINCIPLES OF FIRST AID

1-50. Proper conduct at the initial encounter of the casualty coupled with appropriate movement and transport is important in the successful provision of first aid. Appropriate decisions and first aid task execution helps to determine the health and well-being of the casualty.

INITIAL ENCOUNTER

1-51. When a casualty is first encountered it is imperative that the responder quickly and accurately assess what has occurred, determine the nature and extent of injuries and what (if any) first aid measures are appropriate and necessary.

1-52. Accurately assessing the situation is as important for the safety and well-being of the responder as it is for the casualty. For example, if the casualty is being electrocuted the responder must not directly grab the casualty or he too will become a casualty.

TRANSPORTING OR MOVING THE CASUALTY

1-53. Transporting or moving a casualty by Soldiers providing first aid must be carefully considered for a number of reasons. An example of this type of consideration may be based on the casualty having been involved in a motor vehicle crash. When responding to an accident, first aid providers must consider the possibility of injury to the casualty's spine before extracting the casualty from the vehicle. In this situation moving the casualty may be ill advised unless there is an immediate life-threatening situation such as fire, explosion where the casualty may be at risk of greater injury or death unless moved promptly.

1-54. If there is no danger of greater injury to the casualty by leaving them where they are found, first aid responders should render such aid as is necessary and wait for trained medical personnel to arrive. Once medical personnel are on site they can accurately treat the casualty and direct how and when they should be transported or moved. For detailed discussion on transporting and moving casualties refer to Army Techniques Publication (ATP) 4-25.13.

SECTION IV — COMBAT AND OPERATIONAL STRESS REACTION

1-55. One of the most important functions a Soldier performs is taking care of other Soldiers. The whole of the Army is based on teamwork and the inherent worth of every Soldier. Watching, intervening when and where appropriate, and following through in the battle-buddy concept, is critical in dealing with combat and operational stress reactions.

SUPPORT

1-56. The best first aid for Soldiers is caring and observant battle buddies and their leaders. The Army as an institution provides combat and operational stress control support from the Soldier and on up to the highest levels of Army leadership. Soldiers need to identify distressed Soldiers, seek assistance, and support their battle buddies.

GUIDANCE FOR SUPPORTING AT-RISK SOLDIERS

1-57. The Army has developed a tool for Soldiers and leaders to use to provide some guidelines on how to approach a distressed Soldier. You should—

- Ask.
- Care.
- Escort.

ASK

1-58. Ask your buddy how he is doing and whether or not he feels suicidal. The best way to ask someone if he is suicidal is to do just that. Ask the question: Are you suicidal? It is that simple.

CARE

1-59. Care for your buddy. Upon recognition that your buddy is feeling suicidal, calmly remove any weapons or other items that may increase risk. It is extremely important to remain calm, as your anxiety will have an impact on your ability to calm the Soldier. Remaining calm will also increase your effectiveness at intervening. Once any weapon or other potentially dangerous items are removed, be there for the Soldier. Never leave him alone. Remember, we never leave a fallen comrade and these situations are no different.

ESCORT

1-60. Escort the Soldier to get help and assistance, staying at his side. Failure to stay involved can have a devastating impact on the Soldier and his ability to drive on. Failure to act increases the risk of the Soldier ★ impulsively acting on his suicidal intent. Refer to ATP 6-22.5 for more information.

Chapter 2
Evaluate a Casualty (081-COM-1001)

2-1. Evaluation of a casualty is necessary to identify and treat all life-threatening conditions and other serious wounds. Rapid and accurate evaluation of the casualty is the key to providing effective first aid.

WARNING

If a broken neck or back is suspected, do not move the casualty unless to save his life.

CARE UNDER FIRE

2-2. Performing care under fire—

- Return fire as directed or required before providing first aid.
- Determine if the casualty is alive or dead.

Note. In combat, the most likely threat to the casualty's life is from bleeding. Attempts to check for airway and breathing will expose the rescuer to enemy fire. DO NOT attempt to provide first aid when your own life is in imminent danger. In a combat situation, if you find a casualty with no signs of life, no pulse, no breathing, DO NOT attempt to restore the airway. DO NOT continue first aid measures.

- Provide care to the living casualty. Direct the casualty to return fire, move to cover, and administer self-aid (stop bleeding), if possible.

Note. Reducing or eliminating enemy fire may be more important to the casualty's survival than the treatment you can provide. If the casualty is unable to move and you are unable to move the casualty to cover and the casualty is still under direct enemy fire, have the casualty *play dead.*

- Once enemy fire has been suppressed, conduct the following:
  - In a battle-buddy team, approach the casualty (use smoke or other concealment if available) using the most direct route possible.
  - Administer lifesaving hemorrhage control.
  - Determine the relative threat of enemy fire versus the risk of the casualty bleeding to death.
  - If the casualty has severe, life-threatening bleeding from an extremity or has an amputation of an extremity, administer lifesaving hemorrhage control by applying a tourniquet from the casualty's IFAK before moving the casualty. See Chapter 6, Task 081-COM-1032, on page 6-1.

Note. The only treatment that should be given at the point of injury is a tourniquet to control life threatening extremity bleeding.

  - Move the casualty, his weapon, and mission-essential equipment when the tactical situation permits.
  - Recheck bleeding control measures (tourniquet) as soon as behind cover and not under enemy fire.

TACTICAL FIELD CARE

2-3. Once under cover and not under hostile fire, perform tactical field care as follows:

Note. When evaluating and/or treating a casualty, seek medical aid as soon as possible. DO NOT stop first aid. If the situation allows, send another person to find medical aid.

- Form a general impression of the casualty as you approach (extent of injuries, chance of survival).

Note. If a casualty is being burned, take steps to remove the casualty from the source of the burns before continuing evaluation and first aid. See Chapter 7, Task 081-COM-1007, on page 7-1.

- Ask in a loud, but calm, voice: *Are you okay?* Gently shake or tap the casualty on the shoulder.
- Determine the level of consciousness by using the mnemonic AVPU: A = Alert; V = responds to Voice; P = responds to Pain; U = Unresponsive.

Note. To check a casualty's response to pain, rub the breastbone briskly with a knuckle or squeeze the first or second toe over the toenail. If casualty is wearing individual body armor, pinch his nose or his earlobe for responsiveness.

- If the casualty is conscious, ask where his body feels different than usual, or where it hurts.

Note. If the casualty is conscious but is choking and cannot talk, stop the evaluation and begin appropriate first aid. See Chapter 4, Task 081-COM-1003, on page 4-1.

2-4. Identify and control bleeding—

- Check for bleeding as follows:
  - Reassess any tourniquets placed during the care under fire phase to ensure they are still effective.
  - Perform a blood sweep of the extremities, neck, axillary, inguinal, and extremity areas. Exposure is only necessary if bleeding is detected.
  - Place your hands behind the casualty's neck and pass them upward toward the top of the head. Note whether there is blood or brain tissue on your hands from the casualty's wounds.
  - Place your hands behind the casualty's shoulders and pass them downward behind the back, the thighs, and the legs.

Note. Look to see if there is blood on your hands from the casualty's wounds. If life-threatening bleeding is present, stop the evaluation and control the bleeding. See Chapter 6, Task 081-COM-1032, on page 6-1.

- Once bleeding has been controlled, position the casualty and open the airway. See Chapter 3, Task 081-COM-1023, on page 3-1.

2-5. Assess for breathing and chest injuries as follows:

- Expose the chest and check for equal rise and fall and for any wounds.
- Look, listen, and feel for respiration. See Chapter 3, Task 081-COM-1023, on page 3-1.

Note. If the casualty is breathing, insert a nasopharyngeal airway (see Chapter 3, Task 081-COM-1023, on page 3-1) and place the casualty in the recovery position. Only in the case of nontraumatic injuries such as hypothermia, near drowning, or electrocution should cardiopulmonary resuscitation (CPR) be considered when in a tactical environment prior to the tactical evacuation phase.

- If in a nontactical environment, begin rescue breathing as necessary to restore breathing and or pulse. See Chapter 3, Task 081-COM-1023, on page 3-1.
- If the casualty has a penetrating chest wound and is breathing or attempting to breathe, stop the evaluation to apply an occlusive dressing and position or transport with the affected side down, if possible. See Chapter 5, Task 081-COM-1026, on page 5-1.
- Check for an exit wound. If found, apply an occlusive dressing.
- Dress all nonlife-threatening injuries and any bleeding that has not been addressed earlier with appropriate dressings. See Chapter 6, Task 081-COM-1032, on page 6-1.
- Determine the need to evacuate the casualty and supply information for lines 3 to 5 of the 9-line medical evacuation request to your tactical leader. See Soldier Training Publication (STP) 21-1-SMCT, Chapter 3, Task 081-COM-0101, on page 6-1.

2-6. Check the casualty for burns as follows:

- Look carefully for reddened, blistered, or charred skin. Also check for singed clothes.
- If burns are found, stop the evaluation and begin treatment. See Chapter 7, Task 081-COM-1007, on page 7-1.
- Administer pain medications and antibiotics (casualty's combat pill pack) if available.

Note. Each Soldier will be issued a combat pill pack before deploying on tactical missions.

- Document the injuries and the treatment given on the casualty's own DD Form 1380, Tactical Combat Casualty Care (TCCC) Card (found in the IFAK), if applicable.

TACTICAL EVACUATION

2-7. Once the casualty is provided appropriate first aid, initiate the tactical evacuation phase.

2-8. Transport the casualty to the evacuation site. See STP 21-1-SMCT, Chapter 3, Task 081-COM-1046.

2-9. Monitor the patient for shock and treat as appropriate. See Chapter 8, Task 081-COM-1005, on page 8-1. Continually reassess casualty until a medical person arrives or the patient arrives at a military treatment facility.

This page intentionally left blank.

Chapter 3
Open the Airway (081-COM-1023)

SAFELY POSITION THE CASUALTY TO OPEN THE AIRWAY

3-1. Techniques to safely position an adult casualty who is unconscious and does not appear to be breathing include the following:

> **WARNING**
>
> **The casualty should be carefully rolled as a whole, so the body does not twist.**

- Roll the casualty onto his back, if necessary, and place him on a hard, flat surface.
- Kneel beside the casualty.
- Raise the near arm and straighten it out above the head.
- Adjust the legs so they are together and straight or nearly straight.
- Place one hand on the back of the casualty's head and neck.
- Grasp the casualty under the arm with the free hand.
- Pull steadily and evenly toward yourself, keeping the head and neck in line with the torso.
- Roll the casualty as a single unit.
- Place the casualty's arms at his sides.

OPENING THE AIRWAY

3-2. If foreign material or vomit is in the mouth, remove it as quickly as possible.

HEAD-TILT CHIN-LIFT METHOD

3-3. To open the airway using the head-tilt chin-lift method—

> **CAUTION**
>
> **DO NOT** use this method if a spinal or neck injury is suspected.

- Kneel at the level of the casualty's shoulders.
- Place one hand on the casualty's forehead and apply firm, backward pressure with the palm to tilt the head back.
- Place the fingertips of the other hand under the bony part of the lower jaw and lift, bringing the chin forward.
- Do not use the thumb to lift.
- Do not completely close the casualty's mouth.
- Do not press deeply into the soft tissue under the chin with the fingers.

JAW-THRUST METHOD

3-4. To open the airway using the jaw thrust method—

Note. Use this method if a spinal or neck injury is suspected. If you are unable to maintain an airway after the second attempt, use the head-tilt chin-lift method. Do not tilt or rotate the casualty's head.

- Kneel above the casualty's head (looking toward the casualty's feet).
- Rest your elbows on the ground or floor.
- Place one hand on each side of the casualty's lower jaw at the angle of the jaw, below the ears.
- Stabilize the casualty's head with your forearms.
- Use the index fingers to push the angles of the casualty's lower jaw forward.

Note. If the casualty's lips are still closed after the jaw has been moved forward, use your thumbs to retract the lower lip and allow air to enter the casualty's mouth.

CHECK FOR BREATHING

3-5. While maintaining the open airway position, place an ear over the casualty's mouth and nose, looking toward the chest and stomach.

- Look for the chest to rise and fall.
- Listen for air escaping during exhalation.
- Feel for the flow of air on the side of your face.
- Count the number of respirations for 15 seconds.
- Take appropriate action.

CAUTION

Do not use the nasopharyngeal airway (NPA) if there is clear fluid (cerebrospinal fluid) coming from the ears or nose. This may indicate a skull fracture.

3-6. If the casualty is unconscious, if respiratory rate is less than 2 in 15 seconds, and/or if the casualty is making snoring or gurgling sounds, insert an NPA.

- Keep the casualty in a face-up position.
- Lubricate the tube of the NPA with water.
- Push the tip of the casualty's nose upward gently.
- Position the tube of the NPA so that the bevel (pointed end) of the NPA faces toward the septum (the partition inside the nose that separates the nostrils). Most NPAs are designed to be placed in the right nostril.

CAUTION

Never force the NPA into the casualty's nostril. If resistance is met, pull the tube out and attempt to insert it in the other nostril. If neither nostril will accommodate the NPA, place the casualty in the recovery position.

- Insert the NPA into the nostril and advance it until the flange rests against the nostril.

- Place the casualty in the recovery position by rolling him as a single unit onto his side, placing the hand of his upper arm under his chin, and flexing his upper leg.
- Watch the casualty closely for life-threatening conditions and check for other injuries, if necessary.

3-7. If the casualty is not breathing, immediately seek medical aid.

3-8. If the casualty resumes breathing at any time during this procedure, the airway should be kept open and the casualty should be monitored. If the casualty continues to breathe, he should be transported to medical aid or medical treatment facility in accordance with the tactical situation.

This page intentionally left blank.

Chapter 4
Airway Obstructions (081-COM-1003)

AIRWAY OBSTRUCTION IDENTIFICATION

4-1. In order for air to flow freely into and out of the lungs, the airway must remain unobstructed. The ability to move air freely can be compromised when a foreign body becomes lodged in the throat (while eating for example).

4-2. The airway may be partially or completely blocked. In either case removing the obstruction is vital. In cases of complete blockage, removing the blockage quickly is critical if the casualty is to survive.

- Determine if the casualty needs help as follows:
  - If a casualty has a mild airway obstruction (able to speak or cough forcefully, may be wheezing between coughs) do not interfere except to encourage the casualty.
  - If the casualty has a severe airway obstruction (poor air exchange and increased breathing difficulty, a silent cough, cyanosis [bluish tinge to the skin], or inability to speak or breathe) continue with abdominal or chest thrusts.

Note. You can ask the casualty one question, *Are you choking*? If the casualty nods yes, help is needed.

- The decision to perform abdominal or chest thrusts is determined by the casualty's condition.

Note. Abdominal thrusts should be used unless the casualty is in advanced stages of pregnancy, is very obese, or has a significant abdominal wound.

ABDOMINAL THRUSTS

Note. Clearing a conscious casualty's airway obstruction can be performed with the casualty either sitting or standing.

4-3. To perform abdominal thrusts—

- Stand behind the casualty.
- Wrap your arms around the casualty's waist.
- Make a fist with one hand.
- Place the thumb side of the fist against the abdomen slightly above the navel and well below the tip of the breastbone.
- Grasp the fist with the other hand.
- Give quick backward and upward thrusts.

Note. Each thrust should be a separate, distinct movement. Thrusts should be continued until the obstruction is expelled or the casualty becomes unconscious.

CHEST THRUSTS

4-4. To perform chest thrusts—

- Stand behind the casualty.
- Wrap your arms under the casualty's armpits and around the chest.

- Make a fist with one hand.
- Give backwards thrusts.

Note. Each thrust should be performed slowly and distinctly with the intent of relieving the obstruction.

- Continue to give abdominal or chest thrusts, as required. Give abdominal or chest thrusts until the obstruction is clear, you are relieved by a qualified person, or the casualty becomes unconscious.

Note. If the casualty becomes unresponsive, lay him down and then start mouth-to-mouth resuscitation procedures.

4-5. If the obstruction is cleared, watch the casualty closely and check for other injuries, if necessary.

4-6. Seek medical aid.

Chapter 5

Perform First Aid for an Open Chest Wound (081-COM-1026)

FIRST AID FOR AN OPEN CHEST WOUND

5-1. First aid procedures for dressing an open chest wound without causing further injury to the casualty include—

- Uncover the wound (unless clothing is stuck to the wound or you are in a chemical environment).

> **CAUTION**
>
> Removing stuck clothing or uncovering the wound in a chemical, biological, radiological, and nuclear environment could cause additional harm.

- If not sure that the wound has penetrated the chest wall completely, treat the wound as though it were an open chest wound. If multiple wounds are found at once, treat the largest one first.
- Place gloved hand or back of hand over open chest wound to create temporary seal.
- Since air can pass through most dressings and bandages, you must seal the open chest wound with a commercial chest seal, plastic, cellophane, or other nonporous, airtight material to prevent air from entering the chest.

5-2. Apply airtight material over the wound as follows:

- Fully open the outer wrapper of the casualty's dressing, commercial chest seal or other airtight material.
- Place the inner surface of the outer wrapper or other airtight material directly over the wound after the casualty exhales completely.
- Ensure that the edges of the airtight material extend 2 inches beyond the edges of the wound.

Note. When applying the airtight material, do not touch the inner surface.

- Apply two inch tape (found in the IFAK) to all four sides of the material securing it to the casualty's chest.

CHECK FOR EXIT WOUND OR OTHER OPEN CHEST INJURIES

5-3. If exit wound or other open chest injuries are found, perform same steps as for entrance wound.

5-4. Apply the casualty's emergency dressing over airtight material.

- Apply the dressing or pad, white side down, directly over the airtight material.
- Have the casualty breathe normally.
- Maintain pressure on the dressing while you wrap the tails (or elastic bandage) around the body and back to the starting point.

- Pass the tail through the plastic pressure device, reverse the tail while applying pressure, continue to wrap the tail around the body, and secure the plastic fastening clip to the last turn of the wrap.
- Ensure that the dressing is secured without interfering with breathing.

POSITION THE CASUALTY

5-5. Place a conscious casualty in the sitting position or on his side (recovery position) with his injured side next to the ground.

Note. If the casualty is having difficulty breathing, place him in a position of comfort to ease breathing.

5-6. Place an unconscious casualty in the recovery position on the injured side.

5-7. Monitor the casualty closely for life-threatening conditions, check for other injuries (if necessary), and treat for shock.

5-8. Seek medical aid.

Chapter 6

Perform First Aid for Bleeding of an Extremity (081-COM-1032)

CONTROL BLEEDING

6-1. When evaluating a casualty it is imperative that an accurate determination be made as to whether the bleeding is life threatening or not. This determination will dictate the methods to be used to control the bleeding.

CAUTION

All body fluids should be considered potentially infectious. Always observe body substance isolation precautions by wearing gloves and eye protection as a minimal standard of protection. In severe cases, you should wear gloves, eye protection, gown and shoe covers to protect yourself from splashes, projectile fluids, spurting fluids or splashes onto your clothing and footwear.

METHODS FOR CONTROLLING EXTERNAL BLEEDING

6-2. There are three methods of controlling external bleeding, they are—

- Direct pressure.
- Pressure dressing.
- Tourniquet.

6-3. If the evaluation determines that the bleeding is life threatening, a tourniquet should be immediately applied.

APPLY DIRECT PRESSURE

6-4. If bleeding is not life threatening, apply direct pressure as follows:

- Expose the wound.
- Place sterile gauze or dressing over the injury site and apply fingertips, palm or entire surface of one hand and apply direct pressure.
- Pack large, gaping wounds with sterile gauze and apply direct pressure.

6-5. Once the bleeding has been controlled, it is important to check a distal pulse to make sure that the dressing has not been applied too tightly. If a pulse is not felt, adjust the dressing to re-establish circulation.

WARNING

The emergency bandage must be loosened if the skin distal to the injury becomes cool, blue, numb, or pulseless.

APPLY A PRESSURE DRESSING

6-6. When applying a bandage always use the casualty's emergency bandage.

- Open the plastic dressing package.
- Apply the dressing, white-side down (sterile, nonadherent pad) directly over the wound.
- Wrap the elastic tail (bandage) around the extremity and run the tail through the plastic pressure bar.
- Reverse the tail while applying pressure and continue to wrap the remainder of the tail around the extremity, while continuing to apply pressure directly over the wound.
- Secure the plastic closure bar to the last turn of the wrap.
- Check the emergency bandage to make sure that it is applied firmly enough to prevent slipping without causing a tourniquet-like effect.

CAUTION

In combat, while under enemy fire, a tourniquet is the primary means to control bleeding. It allows the individual, his battle buddy, or the combat medic to quickly control life threatening hemorrhage until the casualty can be moved away from the firefight. Always treat life threatening hemorrhage while you and the casualty are behind cover.

APPLY A TOURNIQUET

6-7. If the evaluation of the casualty determines that the bleeding is life threatening a commercial tourniquet contained in the IFAK should be immediately applied.

- Pull the free end of the self-adhering band through the buckle and route through the friction adapter buckle.
- Place the tourniquet, 2 to 3 inches above the wound on the injured extremity.
- Pull the self-adhering band tight around the extremity and fasten it back on itself as tightly as possible.
- Twist the windlass until the bleeding stops.
- Lock the windlass in place within the windlass clip.
- Secure the windlass with the windlass strap.
- Assess for absence of a distal pulse.
- Place a *T* and the time of the application on the casualty with a marker.
- Secure the commercial tourniquet in place with tape.

6-8. Once the injuries have been bandaged and the bleeding stopped initiate treatment for shock as needed. See Chapter 8, Task 081-COM-1005, on page 8-1.

6-9. Seek medical aid.

Chapter 7

Perform First Aid for Burns (081-COM-1007)

PERFORM FIRST AID FOR BURNS

7-1. The first course of action when attempting to provide first aid for burns is to remove the casualty from the source of the burn to prevent further harm.

> **CAUTION**
>
> Synthetic materials, such as nylon, may melt and cause further injury.

KINDS OF BURNS

7-2. There are four kinds of burns which are likely to be encountered. They are—

- Thermal burns.
  - Remove the casualty from the source of the burn. If the casualty's clothing is on fire, cover the casualty with a field jacket or any large piece of nonsynthetic material and roll him on the ground to put out the flames.

> **WARNING**
>
> **DO NOT touch the casualty or the electrical source with your bare hands. You will be injured too!**

- Electrical burns.

> **WARNING**
>
> **High voltage electrical burns from an electrical source or lightning may cause temporary unconsciousness, difficulties in breathing, or difficulties with the heart (irregular heartbeat).**

  - If the casualty is in contact with an electrical source, turn the electricity off, if the switch is nearby. If the electricity cannot be turned off, use nonconductive material (rope, clothing, or dry wood) to drag the casualty away from the source.

> **WARNING**
>
> **Blisters caused by a blister agent are actually burns. DO NOT try to decontaminate the skin where blisters have already formed. If blisters have not formed, decontaminate the skin.**

- Chemical burns.

- Remove liquid chemicals from the burned casualty by flushing with as much water as possible.
- Remove dry chemicals by carefully brushing them off with a clean, dry cloth. If large amounts of water are available, flush the area. Otherwise, do not apply water.
- Smother burning white phosphorus with water, a wet cloth, or wet mud. Keep the area covered with wet material.

- Laser burns.
  - Move the casualty away from the source while avoiding eye contact with the beam source.
  - If possible, wear appropriate laser eye protection.

Note. After the casualty has been removed from the source of the burn, continually monitor the casualty for conditions that may require basic lifesaving measures.

WARNING

DO NOT uncover the wound in a chemical, biological, radiological, and nuclear environment. Exposure could cause additional harm.

7-3. Uncover the burn as follows:

WARNING

DO NOT attempt to remove clothing that is stuck to the wound. Additional harm could result.

- Cut clothing from the burned area.

CAUTION

DO NOT pull clothing over the burns.

- Gently lift away clothing covering the burned area.
- If the casualty's hands or wrists have been burned, remove jewelry (rings, watches) and place them in his pockets.

7-4. Apply the casualty's dry, sterile dressing directly over the wound as follows:

Note. If the burn is caused by white phosphorus, the dressing must be wet.

CAUTION

DO NOT place the dressing over the face or genital area.

DO NOT break blisters.

DO NOT apply grease or ointments to the burns.

- Apply the dressing or pad, white-side down, directly over the wound.
- Wrap the tail (or the elastic bandage) so the dressing or pad is covered.
- For a field dressing, tie the tails into a nonslip knot over the outer edge of the dressing, not over the wound. For an emergency bandage, secure the hooking ends of the closure bar into the elastic bandage.
- Check to ensure that the dressing is applied lightly over the burn but firmly enough to prevent slipping.

Note. If the casualty is conscious and not nauseated, give him small amounts of water to drink.

7-5. Watch the casualty closely for signs of life-threatening conditions, check for other injuries (if necessary), and treat for shock.

7-6. Seek medical aid.

This page intentionally left blank.

Chapter 8

Perform First Aid to Prevent or Control Shock (081-COM-1005)

SIGNS AND SYMPTOMS OF SHOCK

8-1. Check the casualty for signs and symptoms of shock.

- Sweaty but cool skin.
- Pale skin.
- Restlessness or nervousness.
- Thirst.
- Severe bleeding.
- Confusion.
- Rapid breathing.
- Blotchy blue skin.
- Nausea and/or vomiting.

POSITION THE CASUALTY

8-2. Procedures for positioning the casualty include—

- Move the casualty under a permanent or improvised shelter to shade him from direct sunlight.
- Lay the casualty on his back unless a sitting position will allow the casualty to breathe easier.
- Elevate the casualty's feet higher than the heart using a stable object so the feet will not fall.

WARNING

Do not loosen clothing if in a chemical area.

- Loosen clothing at the neck, waist, or anywhere it is binding.
- Prevent the casualty from getting chilled or overheated. Using a blanket or clothing, cover the casualty to avoid loss of body heat by wrapping completely around the casualty.

Note. Ensure no part of the casualty is touching the ground, as this increases loss of body heat.

CALM AND REASSURE THE CASUALTY

8-3. Calm and reassure the casualty by—

- Taking charge and show self-confidence.
- Assuring the casualty that he is being taken care of.

8-4. Watch the casualty closely for life-threatening conditions and check for other injuries, if necessary.

8-5. Seek medical aid.

This page intentionally left blank.

Chapter 9

Perform First Aid for Nerve Agent Injury (081-COM-1044)

FIRST AID FOR NERVE AGENT INJURY

9-1. After reacting appropriately to a chemical attack (stop breathing, don your protective mask [see STP 21-1-SMCT, Chapter 3, Task 031-COM-1035]) and giving the alarm, it is important to observe yourself and other Soldiers for signs and symptoms of nerve agent poisoning.

9-2. There are two categories of nerve agent poisoning that Soldiers should be familiar with. These are—

- Mild nerve agent poisoning.
- Severe nerve agent poisoning.

9-3. Accurately determining if the poisoning is mild or severe helps to determine what first aid measures are necessary and appropriate.

9-4. To determine what steps are necessary, it is important to identify if the poisoning is mild or severe in nature. There are signs and symptoms specific to each category of nerve agent poisoning.

SIGNS AND SYMPTOMS OF MILD NERVE AGENT POISONING

9-5. Signs and symptoms of mild nerve agent poisoning include—

- Unexplained runny nose.
- Unexplained sudden headache.
- Sudden drooling.
- Tightness in the chest or difficulty breathing.
- Difficulty seeing (dimness of vision or miosis).
- Localized sweating and muscular twitching in the area of contaminated skin.
- Stomach cramps.
- Nausea.

SELF-AID FOR MILD NERVE AGENT POISONING

9-6. First aid for mild nerve agent poisoning is considered to be self-aid.

9-7. First aid, self-aid for mild nerve agent poisoning involves the use of the antidote treatment nerve agent, autoinjector (ATNAA). Administer the ATNAA as follows:

- Acquire one ATNAA autoinjector.

Note. Administer ONLY one ATNAA as self-aid. DO NOT self-administer the convulsant antidote for nerve agent (CANA).

- Locate injection site (outer thigh muscle, about a hands width below the hip joint and above the knee) and ensure that it is clear of objects that will interfere with the injection.

Note. If the individual is thinly built, injection should be given into the upper outer quadrant of the buttock.

CAUTION

DO NOT cover or hold the needle end with your hand, thumb, or fingers. You may accidently inject yourself.

- With your dominant hand, hold the ATNAA in your closed fist with the needle (green) end extending beyond the little finger in front of you at eye level.
- Pull off the safety cap from the bottom of the injector with a smooth motion using the nondominant hand, and drop it to the ground.

CAUTION

When injecting antidote into the buttock, be very careful to inject only into upper, outer quarter of the buttock to avoid hitting the major nerve that crosses the buttocks. Hitting the nerve may cause paralysis.

- Place the needle end of the injector against chosen injection site and apply firm, even pressure until the needle activates into the muscle.

Note. A jabbing motion is not necessary to trigger the activating mechanism.

- Hold the injector firmly in place for at least 10 seconds.
- Remove the injector from your muscle.
- Secure the used injector.
- Bend the needles of all used injectors by pressing on a hard surface to form a hook.
- Attach all used injectors to a blouse pocket flap or the Joint Service Lightweight Integrated Suit Technology (JSLIST).

WARNING

DO NOT give yourself additional injections. If you are able to walk without assistance and know who you are and where you are, you will NOT need the second set of injections. If you continue to have symptoms of nerve agent poisoning, seek someone else (a buddy) to check your symptoms and administer the additional set of injections, if required.

- Massage the injection site, mission permitting.

SIGNS AND SYMPTOMS OF SEVERE NERVE AGENT POISONING

9-8. Signs and symptoms of severe nerve agent poisoning include—

- Strange or confused behavior.
- Wheezing, difficulty breathing, and coughing.
- Severely pinpointed pupils.
- Red eyes with tearing.
- Vomiting.
- Severe muscular twitching.
- Involuntary urination and defecation.

- Convulsions.
- Unconsciousness with, or without respiratory failure.
- Localized sweating and muscular twitching in the area of contaminated skin.

BUDDY AID FOR SEVERE NERVE AGENT POISONING

9-9. First aid for severe nerve agent poisoning is considered buddy aid, it involves the use of the ATNAA and includes administering the CANA with the third ATNAA to prevent convulsions.

9-10. Administer buddy aid for severe nerve agent poisoning.

- Mask the casualty if necessary.
- If the casualty can follow instructions, have him clear his mask.
- Check for a complete mask seal by covering the inlet valves of the mask.
- Pull the protective hood over the head of the casualty.
- Position the casualty on the right side (recovery position) with the head slanted down so that the casualty will not roll back over.

9-11. Administer ATNAA as follows:

CAUTION

Squat, do not kneel, when masking the casualty or administering the nerve agent antidotes to the casualty.

- Position yourself near the casualty's thigh.
- Obtain the casualty's three or remaining ATNAA auto-injectors.

Note. Be sure to use the casualty's own autoinjectors, and not your own.

- Using the same method as in self-aid, administer up to, but no more than three doses of the ATNAA.

Note. If the casualty's condition improves (regains consciousness, become coherent, able to stand or walk) after the first or second dose, do not administer the remaining dose(s), but monitor until medical help arrives or he is evacuated to a higher role of care.

- Bend the needles of all used injectors by pressing on a hard surface to form a hook.
- Attach all used injectors to blouse pocket flat or JSLIST.

9-12. Administer CANA as follows:

Note. Buddy aid also includes administering the CANA with the third ATNAA to prevent convulsions.

CAUTION

Squat, DO NOT kneel when masking the casualty or administering the nerve agent antidotes to the casualty.

- Position yourself near the casualty's thigh.
- Obtain one CANA autoinjector.
- Locate injection site (outer thigh muscle, about a hand's width below the hip joint and above the knee) and ensure it is clear of objects that will interfere with the injection.

Note. If the individual is thinly built, injection should be given into the upper outer quadrant of the buttock.

CAUTION

DO NOT cover or hold the needle end with your hand, thumb, or fingers. You may accidently inject yourself.

- With your dominant hand, hold the CANA in your closed fist with the needle extending beyond the little finger at eye level.
- Pull off the safety cap from the bottom of the injector with a smooth motion using the nondominant hand, and drop it to the ground.

CAUTION

When injecting antidote in the buttock, be very careful to inject only into the upper, outer quarter of the buttock to avoid hitting the major nerve that crosses the buttocks. Hitting the nerve may cause paralysis.

- Place the needle end of the injector against the chosen injection site and apply firm, even pressure until the needle activates into the muscle.
- Hold the injector firmly in place for at least 10 seconds.
- Remove the injector from the casualty's muscle.
- Secure the used injector.

9-13. Decontaminate the skin if necessary.

Note. Information on this step is covered in STP 21-1-SMCT, Chapter 3, Task 031-COM-1013.

9-14. Put on remaining protective clothing.

Note. Information on this step is covered in STP 21-1-SMCT, Chapter 3, Task 031-COM-1040.

9-15. Seek medical aid.

Chapter 10

First Aid for Bites and Stings (081-833-0072)

10-1. First aid procedures for a casualty with insect bites or stings, without causing further injury involves—

- Exposing the injury site.

Note. Removing clothing, rings, watches, and other constricting items that are in the area of the bite or sting to prevent circulatory impairment in the event swelling of the extremity occurs.

- Determining the type of insect bite or sting.
- Gathering information from the casualty, ask them if they saw what bit or stung them.

> **WARNING**
>
> **Be alert for indicators of the casualty developing anaphylaxis such as hoarseness, a feeling of swelling or a lump in the throat, wheezing, and signs and symptoms of shock.**

- Checking an unconscious casualty for a medical alert bracelet or tag (allergy band).

Note. It is important to determine if the casualty has a history of past reactions to similar bites or stings.

10-2. Assess the casualty for signs and symptoms of insect bites or stings.

BLACK WIDOW SPIDER

10-3. Signs and symptoms of black widow spider bites include—

- A pinprick sensation at the bite site, becoming a dull ache within about 30 minutes.
- Severe painful muscle spasms, especially in the shoulders, back, chest and abdomen.
  - Begin in 10 to 40 minutes.
  - Peak in 1 to 3 hours.
  - Persist for 12 to 48 hours.
- Rigid, board-like abdomen.
- Dizziness, nausea, vomiting, and respiratory distress in severe cases.

10-4. Signs and symptoms of brown recluse spider bites include—

Note. The brown recluse spider is medium-sized, generally brown but can range in color from yellow to dark chocolate brown. It has a distinct groove between its chest and abdominal body parts. The characteristic marking is a brown, violin-shaped marking on the upper back.

- Casualty seldom recalls being bitten, since the bite is painless at first.
- Several hours after the bite, it becomes bluish surrounded by a white periphery.

- A red halo or *bulls-eye* pattern appears sometime later.
- Within 7 to 10 days, the bite becomes a large ulcer.

SCORPION (HARMLESS SPECIES)

10-5. Signs and symptoms of scorpion (harmless species) stings include—

Note. There are two general types of scorpions. The Arizona (black) scorpion is the only deadly type in the United States.

- Severity of the sting depends on the amount of venom injected.
- Ninety percent of all scorpion stings occur on the hands.
- Scorpion stings cause a sharp pain at the injection site.
- The symptoms last for 24 to 72 hours.

SCORPION (DEADLY SPECIES)

10-6. Signs and symptoms of scorpion (deadly species) stings include—

- Sharp pain at the injection site, "pins and needles" sensation.
- Severe muscle contractions.
- Drooling.
- Poor circulation.
- Hypertension.
- Cardiac failure.
- Incontinence.
- Seizures.

BEE, WASP, HORNET, AND YELLOW JACKET (MILD REACTION)

10-7. Signs and symptoms of a mild reaction to bee, wasp, hornet, and yellow jacket stings include—

Note. A wasp or yellow jacket (slender body with elongated abdomen) retains its stinger and can sting repeatedly. A honey bee (round abdomen) usually leaves its stinger in the casualty.

- Pain at the sting site.
- A wheal, redness, and swelling.
- Itching.
- Anxiety.

BEE, WASP, HORNET, AND YELLOW JACKET (SEVERE REACTION)

10-8. Signs and symptoms of a severe reaction to bee, wasp, hornet, and yellow jacket stings include—

- Generalized itching and burning.
- Urticaria (hives).
- Chest tightness and cough.
- Swelling around the lips and tongue.
- Bronchospasm (narrowing of the airways in the lungs) and wheezing.
- Dyspnea (shortness of breath).
- Abdominal cramps.
- Anxiety.

- Respiratory distress.
- Anaphylactic shock.

FIRE ANT STINGS AND BITES

10-9. Signs and symptoms of fire ant bites and stings include—

Note. Fire ants inject a very irritating toxin into the skin. They bite repeatedly and in a very short time. Fire ants are known for their aggressive nature and for their bites. A fire ant sting itches, is painful, and prone to infection.

- Intense, fiery, burning pain.
- Characteristic circular pattern of bites.

Note. Fire ants bite down into the skin, then sting downwardly as they pivot.

- Extremely painful vesicles that are filled with fluid within minutes.
- Cloudy, fluid-filled bubble within 2 to 4 hours.
- Bubble on red base within 8 to 10 hours.
- Ulceration (with scarring after healing).
- Fire ant bites can also cause large local reaction characterized by swelling, pain and redness that affects the entire extremity.
- Anaphylactic shock.

WARNING

Lyme disease, usually transmitted by the tiny deer tick but now thought to be transmitted by the larger dog tick, can cause long-term neurological and other complications if not identified and treated early.

TICKS

Note. Tick bites are serious because ticks can carry tick fever, Rocky Mountain spotted fever, Lyme disease, other bacterial diseases, and may even cause anemia if the infestation is severe enough.

10-10. Signs and symptoms of tick bites include—

- Itching and redness at the site.
- Headache.
- Moderate to high fever, which may last 2 to 3 weeks.
- Pain in the joints or legs.
- Swollen lymph nodes in the bitten area.

CAUTION

Generally, a tick must remain attached to the body for 4 to 6 hours in order to transmit infections. Early detection and proper removal may prevent transmission.

- Paralysis and other central nervous system disorders are possible after several days.

UNKNOWN, NONSPECIFIC INSECTS

10-11. Signs and Symptoms of unknown, nonspecific insects include—

- Pain and swelling at the site.
- Breathing difficulty.
- Shock.

> **WARNING**
>
> **If the casualty shows signs and symptoms of an allergic reaction, begin transport immediately.**

TREAT THE BITE OR STING

10-12. Treat black widow spider, brown recluse, fire ant, and scorpion bites and stings as follows:

- Keep the casualty calm and reassured.
- Explain to the casualty what will be done.
- Limit their physical activity.

Note. Keep the body immobilized and the casualty still to prevent distribution of the poison to other parts of the body.

- Remove jewelry.
- Cleanse the bite site gently using normal saline (or cleanest water available) and mild or strong soap solution.

Note. If necessary, irrigate the area with large amount of sterile saline (or the cleanest water available). Make sure that the contaminated saline (clean water) flows away from the body. Never scrub the area.

> **CAUTION**
>
> Application of cold packs to insect bite or sting to relieve pain and swelling should be followed in accordance with local standard operating procedures and medical officer's order.

- Apply a cold pack to an insect bite or sting to relieve pain and swelling.
- Treat the casualty for anaphylactic shock, if necessary. See STP 8-68W13-SM-TG, Chapter 3, Task 081-833-0003.
- Monitor vital signs.
- Seek medical aid.

10-13. Treat tick bites as follows:

- Remove all parts of the tick.
- Using tweezers, grasp the tick as close to the skin as possible. Using steady pressure, pull the tick straight out.
- If tweezers are not available, use an absorbent material (gauze, toweling) to protect your skin. Grasp the tick as close to the skin as possible and pull straight out using steady pressure.
- Wash the area around the bite gently using normal saline (or cleanest water available) and a mild or strong soap solution.

- Monitor vital signs.
- Seek medical aid.

10-14. Treat unknown, nonspecific insect as follows:

- Cleanse the site using antiseptic.
- Treat the casualty for anaphylactic shock, if necessary. See STP 8-68W13-SM-TG, Chapter 3, Task 081-833-0003.
- Seek medical aid.

This page intentionally left blank.

Chapter 11
First Aid for Heat Illness (081-831-0038)

HEAT ILLNESS

11-1. Exertional heat illness refers to a spectrum of disorders (for example— cramps, heat exhaustion, heat injury, heat stroke) resulting from total body heat stress. See ATP 4-25.12 and TC 4-02.3 for more information on heat illness.

11-2. While there is a range of adverse effects that can result from the body overheating, the two major kinds of heat illnesses that are referred to as heat casualties are—

- Heat exhaustion (can be mild or more severe).
- Heat stroke (most severe form of heat illness and possibly fatal).

***Note*.** For more information on heat illness prevention, see United States Army Public Health Command Web site.

HEAT EXHAUSTION

11-3. Heat exhaustion is often preceded by heat cramps, muscle cramps of the arms, legs, or abdomen. Heat cramps and heat exhaustion often act as *canaries in the coal mine.* These conditions need to be identified and treated before they get to a more extreme case of heat stroke. Catch these conditions early as casualty needs rest, water, shade, evaluation, and possible medical care.

SIGNS AND SYMPTOMS OF HEAT EXHAUSTION

11-4. Signs and symptoms of heat exhaustion include—

- Dizziness.
- Headache.
- Loss of appetite.
- Nausea.
- Weakness.
- Clumsy/unsteady walk.
- Profuse sweating and pale (or gray), moist cool skin.
- Normal to slightly elevated body temperature.
- Muscle cramps.
- Heat cramps.

FIRST AID FOR HEAT EXHAUSTION

11-5. First aid measures for heat exhaustion include—

- Rest Soldier in shade.
- Loosen uniform and remove head gear.
- Have Soldier drink 2 quarts of water over 1 hour.
- Seek medical aid.
- Evacuate if no improvement in 30 minutes, or if Soldier's condition worsens.

11-6. First aid for heat cramps is the same for heat exhaustion; the goal is to prevent the heat cramps from progressing into heat exhaustion with further complications.

HEAT STROKE

11-7. Heat stroke is a medical emergency and can be fatal if not immediately addressed. The casualty must be evacuated to the nearest medical treatment facility as soon as possible.

SIGNS AND SYMPTOMS HEAT STROKE

11-8. Signs and symptoms for heat stroke include—

- Hot dry skin.
- Headache.

Note. In the early progression of heat stroke, the skin may be moist or wet

---

- Convulsions and chills.
- Dizziness.
- Nausea.
- Weakness.
- Pulse and respirations are weak and rapid
- Vomiting.
- Confusion, mumbling (do mental check questions to see if brain is working correctly).
- Combative.
- Passing out (unconscious).

FIRST AID FOR HEAT STROKE

11-9. Immediately begin cooling the Soldier off (the faster the body is cooled, the less damage to the brain and organs) as follows:

- Cool the casualty with any means available, even before removing clothes.
- Strip (if possible, ensure a same gender helper is present).
- Rapidly cool by immersing the casualty in cold water.
- Rapidly cool with ice sheets as follows:
  - Cover all but face with iced sheets.
  - Ensure the iced sheet is soaked prior to applying to the casualty.
- Place ice packs, if available, in groin, axillae (armpits) and around the neck.
- Fan the entire body.
- Stop cooling if casualty starts shivering.
- Seek medical aid.
- Evacuate immediately, and continue cooling during transport.
- Give nothing by mouth.

Note. The same person should observe the Soldier during cooling and evacuation in order to spot symptom changes.

HYPONATREMIA (WATER INTOXICATION)

11-10. Hyponatremia is a medical emergency which can be mistaken for heat stroke, though treatment is very different.

Note. This condition most often occurs during initial entry training; however, it may occur anytime overhydration is encountered.

SIGNS AND SYMPTOMS OF HYPONATREMIA

11-11. Signs and symptoms for hyponatremia include—

- Mental status changes.
- Vomiting.
- History of consumption of large volume of water.
- Poor food intake.
- Abdomen distended/bloated.
- Large amounts of clear urine.

FIRST AID FOR HYPONATREMIA

11-12. First aid measures for hyponatremia include—

- Do not give more water or intravenous fluids.
- If awake, allow Soldier to consume salty foods or snacks.
- Seek medical aid.
- Evacuate immediately.

This page intentionally left blank.

Chapter 12

First Aid for Cold Injury (081-831-0039)

COLD WEATHER INJURIES

12-1. Cold weather-related injuries include injuries due to decreased temperature (hypothermia, frostbite, and nonfreezing cold injury); injuries due to heaters; carbon monoxide poisoning; and accidents due to impaired physical and/or mental function resulting from cold stress. Cold weather injuries can also occur in warmer ambient temperatures when an individual is wet due to rain or water immersion. For more information, see the United States Army Public Health Command (Cold Weather Casualties and Injuries) Web site. More information concerning cold weather injuries can also be found in ATP 4-25.12 and TC 4-02.3.

HYPOTHERMIA

12-2. Hypothermia is defined as a body core temperature below 95° Fahrenheit (F). Hypothermia is usually characterized as mild, moderate, or severe, based on body core temperature. In order to properly diagnose hypothermia, core temperature must be measured rectally with a thermometer with an extended low range scale. Oral and tympanic temperatures will not yield accurate results in a cold environment, even when care is taken to use the best technique.

> **CAUTION**
>
> Hypothermia is a medical emergency, appropriate first aid and evacuation to the nearest medical treatment facility must be initiated as soon as possible. With generalized hypothermia, the entire body has cooled with the core temperature below 95°F.

12-3. Hypothermia occurs when heat loss is greater than heat production. This can occur suddenly, such as during partial or total immersion in cold water, or over hours or days, such as during extended operations or survival situations.

12-4. Hypothermia may occur at temperatures above freezing, especially when a person's skin or clothing is wet.

SIGNS AND SYMPTOMS OF HYPOTHERMIA

12-5. Signs and symptoms of hypothermia include—

- Vigorous shivering is typically present.
- Shivering may decrease or cease as core temperature continues to fall.
- Conscious, but usually apathetic or lethargic.
- Confusion.
- Sleepiness.
- Slurred speech.
- Shallow breathing.
- Very slow respirations.
- Weak pulse.
- Low or unattainable blood pressure.

- Change in behavior with or without poor control over body movements with or without slow reactions.
- With severe hypothermia, the casualty may be unconscious or stuporous.

First Aid for Hypothermia

12-6. The goals for field management of hypothermia are to rescue, examine, insulate, and rapidly transport. If untreated, hypothermia is a true medical emergency and requires evacuation.

> **CAUTION**
>
> Do not allow the casualty to use tobacco, or consume alcohol or caffeinated drinks.

12-7. Rewarming techniques include—

- Remove the casualty from the cold environment.
- Replace wet clothing with dry clothing.
- Cover the casualty with insulating material or blanket.
- Wrap the casualty from head to toe.
- Avoid unnecessary movement from the casualty.
- If casualty is conscious, slowly give high caloric sweet warm fluids.
- Seek medical aid.
- Evacuate as soon as possible with the casualty lying down.

FROSTBITE

12-8. Frostbite accounts for the largest number of cold weather injuries each year and occurs when tissue is exposed to temperatures that are usually below 32°F depending upon windchill factor, length of exposure, and adequacy of protection.

12-9. Frostbite can occur suddenly due to contact to cold metal or super-cooled liquids such as alcohol, fuel, or antifreeze or can develop over time due to prolonged cold exposure. Frostbite is most common in exposed skin such as the nose, ears, cheeks, but can also occur in the hands and feet due to reduced skin blood flow.

Note. The onset is signaled by a sudden blanching of the skin of the nose, ears, cheeks, fingers, or toes followed by a momentary tingling sensation. Frostbite is indicated when the face, hands, or feet stop hurting.

Signs and Symptoms of Frostbite

12-10. Signs and symptoms of frostbite include—

- Numbness in affected area.
- Tingling, blistered, swollen, or tender areas.
- Pale, yellowish, waxy-looking skin (grayish in dark-skinned soldiers).
- Frozen tissue that feels wooden to the touch.
- Significant pain after rewarming

12-11. The most significant frostbite injury involves—

- Frozen tissue involving full thickness of skin with muscle and bone involvement.
- Necrotic (dead) tissue develops along with sloughing of tissue and autoamputation of nonviable tissue.
- These casualties will have permanent disability.

FIRST AID FOR FROSTBITE

> **CAUTION**
>
> Avoid thawing the affected area if it is possible that the injury may refreeze before reaching the medical treatment facility.

12-12. First aid measures for frostbite include—

- Local rewarming at room temperature or using body heat.
- Loosen or remove constricting clothing and remove jewelry.

> **CAUTION**
>
> DO NOT massage the skin or rub anything on the frozen parts.

- Move the casualty to a sheltered area, if possible.
- Protect the affected area from further cold or trauma.
- Once a tissue is thawed, it must not freeze again. If there is the possibility of tissue refreezing, it is better not to thaw it in order to avoid damaging tissue further.
- Avoid exposure to excessive heat (open flame, stove tops, steam, heat packs) or rubbing affected tissue.
- All Soldiers with a peripheral freezing injury must be suspected of being hypothermic and treated appropriately. During field management, it is more important to prevent hypothermia than to rewarm frostbite rapidly.
- Seek medical aid.
- Evacuate the casualty.

CAUSE OF NONFREEZING COLD INJURIES

12-13. Exposure to temperatures from 32° to 60°F may cause nonfreezing cold injuries of skin, fingers, toes, ears and facial parts.

12-14. Exposure of skin to cold metal; super cold fuel, petroleum, oil, and lubricants; windchill; and the wear of tight, circulation-restricting clothing (particularly boots).

12-15. Riding in open vehicles, exposure to propeller/rotor-generated wind, running or skiing, and altitude exposure where there is little tree cover can all contribute to greater windchill.

MOST COMMON NONFREEZING INJURIES

12-16. Nonfreezing cold injuries are chilblain, snow blindness, and immersion syndrome (immersion foot, trench foot and hand). Trench foot occurs when tissues are exposed to temperatures from 32° to 60°F for prolonged periods of time (>12 hours), whereas chilblains, which is a more superficial injury, can occur after repeated prolonged exposure of bare skin to low temperatures from 60°F down to 32°F. Snow blindness is caused by unprotected exposure to ultraviolet rays. Snow blindness can be prevented by the use of appropriate eye protection (sunglasses). Snow blindness can be painful as late as 3 to 5 hours later.

CHILBLAIN

12-17. Chilblain is a nonfreezing cold weather injury that can occur after 1 to 5 hours in cold, wet conditions at temperatures from about 50°F down to 32°F. The most commonly affected areas are the fingernail-side of the fingers, but the ears, face, and other exposed skin are also areas of occurrence. There are no lasting effects from chilblain.

Signs and Symptoms of Chilblain

12-18. Signs and symptoms of chilblain include—

- Chilblain lesions are swollen, tender, itchy and painful.
- Skin becomes swollen, red (or darkening of the skin in dark-skinned Soldiers) and hot to the touch with rewarming.
- An itching or burning sensation may continue for several hours after exposure.

Note. Early diagnosis of chilblain becomes evident when symptoms do not resolve with rewarming.

First Aid for Chilblain

12-19. Rewarm affected area, keep warm and dry.

IMMERSION FOOT (TRENCH FOOT)

12-20. Like chilblain, immersion syndrome of the feet is a nonfreezing cold-weather injury that can occur in damp, wet conditions. The most commonly affected area is the feet and occasionally involves the hands. If left untreated, or allowed to fester (to become septic), loss of tissue to include loss of limbs and gangrene can result. Permanent disability may result from severe immersion syndrome of the feet or hands.

Signs and Symptoms of Immersion Foot

12-21. Signs and symptoms of immersion foot include—

- Cold, numb feet that may progress to hot with shooting pains.
- Slight sensory change for 2 to 3 days.
- Swelling, redness, and bleeding may become pale and blue.
- Accompanied by aches, increased pain sensitivity and infection.
- Loss of sensation.
- Severe edema and gangrene.
- Loss of tissue.

First Aid for Immersion Foot

12-22. First aid measures for immersion foot include—

- Remove wet or constrictive clothing, gently wash and dry affected extremities.
- Elevate affected limbs and cover with layers of loose, warm, dry clothing.
- Do not pop blisters, apply lotions or creams, massage, expose to extreme heat or permit Soldiers to walk, which can increase tissue damage and worsen the injury.
- Seek medical attention.
- Evacuate for medical treatment.

SNOW BLINDNESS

12-23. Snow blindness in the field is usually caused by Soldiers being exposed to high levels of ultraviolet rays over a period of time without wearing appropriate eye protection such as sunglasses. Pain results after a few hours of exposure and resolves over a period of a day or two. Pain may also be caused by exposure to ultraviolet rays from artificial sources (for example welding machine) in much shorter time.

Signs and Symptoms of Snow Blindness

12-24. Signs and symptoms of snow blindness include—

- Scratchy feeling in the eyes as if from sand or dirt.
- Watery eyes.
- Pain, possibly as late as 3 to 5 hours later.
- Reluctant or unable to open eyes.

First Aid for Snow Blindness

12-25. First aid measures for snow blindness include—

- Cover the eyes with a dark cloth.
- Evacuate the casualty to a medical treatment facility.

This page intentionally left blank.

Chapter 13

Apply a Rigid Splint (081-833-0263)

FRACTURES

13-1. A fracture is a break in the continuity of a bone. When properly cared for fractures generally heal without complication. However if severe enough and improperly cared for they can cause disability, loss of the limb or in some cases death by severing vital organs and/or arteries.

13-2. The potential for recovery depends greatly upon the first aid the individual receives before he is moved. First aid includes immobilizing the fractured part in addition to applying lifesaving measures when necessary. The basic splinting principle is to immobilize the joints above and below the fracture.

13-3. There are two kinds of fractures as follows:

- Closed fracture—is a broken bone that does not break the overlying skin.

Note. Dislocations is when a joint, such as a knee, ankle, or shoulder is not in proper position. A sprain is when the connecting tissues of the joints have been torn. Dislocations and sprains (swelling, possible deformity, and discoloration) should be treated as closed fractures.

- Open fracture—is the result of a broken bone that breaks (pierces) the overlying skin. The broken bone may come through the skin or a missile such as a bullet or shell fragment may go through the flesh and break the bone.

Note. An open fracture is contaminated and subject to infection.

13-4. Signs and symptoms commonly associated with fractures include—

- Deformity.
- Tenderness.
- Swelling.
- Pain.
- Inability to move the injured part.
- Protruding bone.
- Bleeding.
- Discolored skin at the injury site.

13-5. First aid for fractures involves immobilizing the affected area

APPLY A RIGID SPLINT

13-6. After the casualty's other more serious injuries have been assessed and treated, the casualty's suspected fracture of an arm or leg is treated. You will need a rigid or formable splint, four muslin bandages (cravats), three inch tape and a six inch elastic bandage, or field expedient materials in order to apply the rigid splint.

13-7. The splint must immobilize the suspected fracture so it does not move and circulation is not impaired. Take body substance isolation precautions (use the gloves in the IFAK). Prepare the casualty for the application of the splint.

Upper Extremity Fractures

13-8. To splint an upper extremity fracture—

- Have the casualty sit up.
- Have someone support the fractured extremity.
- Remove all jewelry from the fractured extremity.
- Expose the fracture site.

Lower Extremity Fractures

13-9. To splint an lower extremity fracture—

- Have the casualty sit or lie down.
- Have another person manually immobilize the fractured extremity.
- Remove the foot gear and expose the fracture site.

> **WARNING**
>
> **If a pulse cannot be felt, apply gentle manual traction in line with the long axis of the limb. This maneuver may restore the pulse. If a pulse does not return after one attempt, splint the limb in the most comfortable position for the casualty and evacuate the casualty immediately.**

- Check distal (at the wrist) pulse and capillary refill on the injured extremity. Prepare the splint for application.

Note. If using a formable splint, measure and shape the splint on the injured extremity.

Forearm and Wrist Fractures

13-10. To splint a fractured wrist—

- Fold the formable splint in half, upon itself creating a double layered splint, leaving one side approximately 1 inch longer than the other.
- Take the folded end of the formable splint and roll at least two times toward the side with the shortest end. This will provide a natural curvature for the hand when the splint is applied.
- Shape the formable splint into a C curve along the long axis from the rolled end to the opposite end.
- Shape the splint until the splint generally conforms to the curve and shape of the limb being splinted.
- Pad the splint and fill in the voids as needed.
- Place the fractured forearm in the splint with the hand in a natural curve on top of the rolled end of the splint.
- Tie one cravat above (proximal) and one cravat below (distal) the fracture site.
- Tie the tails of the cravats in a nonslip knot on the outside of the splint.
- Recheck the casualty's pulse (at the wrist) and capillary refill. Loosen the cravats and reapply the splint if needed.
- Cut the tails of the each cravat to prevent accidental entanglement when the casualty is moved.
- Apply a sling and a swath to further immobilize the fractured arm. See Chapter 20, Task 081-833-0265, on page 20-1.

Elbow Injury

13-11. To splint an injured elbow—

- The injured extremity should be placed in a V (bent) position with the forearm across the front of the chest between the neck and the abdomen (anterior thorax).
- Take one splint and fold in half, fold the splint in half again but along the long axis of the splint.
- Pad the formable splint if needed.

Fractured Long-Bone of the Arm (Humerus)

13-12. To splint a fractured long-bone of the arm—

- Fold one third of the 36 inch formable splint upon itself to create a 12 inch section of double-layered splint.
- Bend the double layered portion of the splint into a J and tape both layers together.
- Support the casualty's arm in an L shape.
- Hook the elbow with the J portion of the splint, running the rest of the splint along the upper arm towards the shoulder (on the outside of the arm).
- Fold any excess splint that may be extending above the top of the shoulder, back upon itself (double layer).
- Secure the splint with an elastic bandage below and above and then secure the elastic bandage with tape.
- Apply a sling and swathe to further immobilize the fractured arm. See Chapter 20, Task 081-833-0265, on page 20-1.

LOWER EXTREMITY INJURY

13-13. To splint an lower extremity fracture—

- Have the casualty sit or lie down.
- Have another person manually immobilize the fractured extremity.
- Remove the foot gear and expose the fracture site.

Ankle Injury

13-14. To splint an injured ankle—

- Apply padding to the bony prominence of the medial and lateral ankle bones (middle to outside portion of the ankles).
- Fold a 36 inch formable splint to create two equal halves.

Note. When folding a formable splint, make sure the middle fold is large enough to accommodate the foot.

- Fold both sides of the splint in a slight C to create rigidity along the long axis of the splint.
- Apply the splint to the ankle by placing the foot in the stirrup position of the splint.
- Form the splint to the length of the lower leg.
- Secure the splint by wrapping the elastic bandage from the top of the foot around the bottom of the foot and up the length of the splint.
- Tape the wrap in place.

Tibula and or Fibula Fracture (Bones of the Lower Leg)

13-15. To splint an injured tibula and or fibula—

- Apply padding to the bony prominence of the medial and lateral ankle bones (across the middle and outside of the ankle bones).
- Completely extend the entire 36 inch formable splint.
- Curve approximately six inches of the splint into a J shape.
- Form a C curve along the long axis of the remaining 30 inches of the splint.
- Perform the same steps to another 36 inches formable splint.
- Apply the splint to the outside area of the fractured tibia/fibula.
- Place the foot in the J portion of the splint and run the long axis of the splint up the leg toward the knee.
- Wrap both splints around the lower leg with an elastic bandage starting from the top of the foot, around the bottom of the foot and then up the length of the splints toward the knee.
- Apply the second splint to the inside area of the fractured tibia/fibula.
- Place the foot (with the previous splint) into the J and run the long axis of the splint up the leg toward the knee.
- Tape the wrap in place.
- Recheck the distal (at the ankle) pulse.

Prepare Cravats

Note. If cravats are to be used in securing the splint to the injured extremity, position the cravats above and below the fracture site.

13-16. Apply and secure the splint to the injured extremity with the limb in the position of function.

Fractures of the Femur

13-17. When a casualty has a fractured femur he should not be moved unless leaving him in place would result in greater injury being inflicted. Never attempt to straighten or apply traction on the fractured limb. Leave that procedure to medical personnel.

CAUTION

A fractured femur is a medical emergency. Medical assistance must be sought as soon as possible. Moving the casualty with a fractured femur may cause further life-threatening injury. If the casualty must be moved, ensure that the utmost care is taken when moving the casualty.

13-18. When applying board splints to the long bones, ensure they are padded sufficiently over the boney parts of the leg.

13-19. Cravats are placed above and below the fracture.

13-20. An anatomical splint may be used, using the uninjured leg as the splint. Ensure the cravats, belts and other appropriate materials hold the leg security above and below the fracture as well as at the feet.

13-21. Poles rolled in blanket and used as splints and tied off with cravats above and below the fracture site. The two cravats or other suitable material cover the chest and abdomen to secure the splint to the torso. Another cravat to hold the splint to the upper leg above the fracture and a minimum of three cravats below the fracture site.

13-22. Observe for shock and apply first aid measures if necessary. See Chapter 8, Task 081-COM-1005, on page 8-1.

Note. Recheck the distal pulse (anatomical point away from the injury) periodically to ensure that the swelling has not compromised the extremity. If swelling occurs and the distal pulse is lost, evacuate the casualty immediately.

13-23. Record treatment given on the TCCC Card (DD Form 1380).

13-24. Seek medical assistance and evacuate the casualty as soon as possible.

This page intentionally left blank.

Chapter 14

Rescue Breathing (081-831-0048)

PERFORM RESCUE BREATHING

14-1. If the casualty does not promptly resume adequate spontaneous breathing after the airway is open, rescue breathing (artificial respiration) must be started as follows:

- Position yourself at the side or directly above the casualty's head.
- Open the airway. See Chapter 3, Task 081-COM-1023, on page 3-1.
- Use the head-tilt chin-lift method when there is no suspected spinal injury.

> **WARNING**
>
> **Foreign body airway obstructions such as those caused by food or small objects are difficult to see and can cause both partial and complete airway obstructions.**

- Use the jaw thrust maneuver when trauma is observed or there is a suspected spinal injury.

Note. Several factors can make it difficult to establish a patent airway such as trauma to the face that causes swelling and bleeding making it difficult to keep the airway clear.

- Ventilate the casualty using the mouth-to-mouth or mouth-to-nose, as appropriate.

MOUTH-TO-MOUTH METHOD

14-2. Perform the mouth-to-mouth method of rescue breathing as follows:

- Maintain the chin-lift method while pinching the nostrils closed using the thumb and index fingers of your hand on the casualty's forehead.
- Take a regular breath and make an airtight seal around the casualty's mouth with your mouth.
- Give one slow breath (lasting one second) into the casualty's mouth, watching for the chest to rise and fall and listening and feeling for air to escape upon your cheek.

Note. You must let go of the casualty's nose once you have given the breath and you are watching for the rise and fall of the chest, in order to feel the air escape upon your cheek.

- If the chest rises and air escapes give a second slow breath.

14-3. Check the carotid pulse, for at least five seconds but no longer than 10 seconds as follows:

- While maintaining the airway, place the index and middle fingers of your hand on the casualty's throat.
- Slide the fingers into the groove beside the casualty's Adam's apple and feel for a pulse for no longer than 10 seconds.
- If a pulse is present, continue rescue breathing at the following rate:
  - Adults: 12 to 20 breaths per minute.
  - Children (one year of age to onset of puberty): 15 to 30 breaths per minute.
  - Infants (less than one year of age): 25 to 50 breaths per minute.

- Watch for rising and fall of chest.
- If a pulse is not found, initiate CPR. See Chapter 15, Task 081-831-0046, on page 15-1.
- If the chest does not rise or air does not escape, reposition the head, and repeat. Give a second slow breath and check the carotid pulse.

MOUTH-TO-NOSE METHOD

14-4. The mouth-to-nose method is recommended when you cannot open the casualty's mouth, there are mouth or jaw injuries, or you cannot maintain a tight seal around the casualty's mouth.

14-5. Initiate mouth-to-nose breathing as follows:

- Maintain the head-tilt with the hand on the forehead while using the other hand to lift the casualty's jaw and close the mouth.
- Take a regular breath and make an airtight seal around the casualty's nose with your mouth.
- Blow one full breath (lasting one second) into the casualty's nose with your mouth.

Note. It may be necessary to open the casualty's mouth, or to separate the lips to allow air to escape.

- If the chest rises give a second full breath.
- Check the carotid pulse for at least five seconds but no longer than 10 seconds. While maintaining the airway, place the index and middle fingers of your hand on the casualty's throat. Slide your fingers into the groove beside the casualty's Adam's apple and feel for a pulse no longer than 10 seconds.
- If a pulse is present, continue rescue breathing at the following rate:
  - Adults: 12 to 20 breaths per minute.
  - Children (one year of age to onset of puberty): 15 to 30 breaths per minute.
  - Infants (less than one year of age): 25 to 50 breaths per minute.
- Watch for rising and falling of the chest.

14-6. If a pulse is not found, initiate CPR and seek medical aid. See Chapter 15, Task 081-831-0046, on page 15-1.

Chapter 15

External Chest Compressions (081-831-0046)

15-1. When coming upon an unresponsive, pulseless casualty who also exhibits a temporary interruption of breathing, time is of the essence in providing effective CPR. Administer external chest compressions until pulse is restored, you are relieved by other competent personnel, too exhausted to continue, the casualty is pronounced dead by an authorized person, or enemy fire prevents you from continuing until the casualty is moved behind cover.

15-2. Establish unresponsiveness (gently shake the casualty, asking, *Are you OK?*).

- Assess the casualty for a response and look for normal or abnormal breathing.

Note. If there is no response and no breathing or no normal breathing (for example only gasping) shout for help.

- Tap the casualty's shoulder and shout, *Are you all right?*
- If the casualty is **unresponsive**, ***activate the emergency response system!*** This is typically accomplished by calling 911.
- If responsive, continue evaluating the casualty.

15-3. Check for signs of circulation as follows:

- Attempt to feel the casualty's carotid pulse (do not take more than 10 seconds).
- If the casualty has a carotid pulse but is not breathing, perform rescue breathing. See Chapter 14, Task 081-0831-0048, on page 14-1.
- If you do not definitely feel a pulse within 10 seconds, perform 5 cycles of compressions and breaths (30:2 ratio) starting with compressions (compressions-airway-breathing sequence).

15-4. Begin chest compressions as follows:

- Ensure that the casualty is positioned on a hard, flat surface, in a supine position. Kneel next to the casualty.

Note. If you suspect the casualty has a head or neck injury, try to keep the head, neck and torso in line when rolling the casualty to a face up position.

- Position yourself on the casualty's side.
- Place the heel of one hand on the center of the casualty's chest on the lower half of the breastbone.

Note. You may either extend or interlace your fingers but keep your fingers off the casualty's chest.

- Place the heel of your other hand on top of the first hand.
- Straighten your arms and lock your elbows and position your shoulders directly over your hands.
- Give 30 compressions.
- Push hard and fast.
- Press down at least 2 inches (5 centimeters) with each compression.

Note. For each chest compression, make sure you push straight down on the casualty's breast bone. This will require hard work. Adequate depth must be attained for at least 23 of the 30 compressions.

- Deliver compressions in a smooth fashion at the rate of 100 per minute, (for example, an adequate rate would be 30 compressions in 18 seconds of less).
- At the end of each compression, make sure you allow the chest to recoil (re-expand) completely.

CAUTION

DO NOT move the casualty with CPR in progress unless the casualty is in a dangerous environment, or if you cannot perform CPR effectively in the casualty's present position or location.

- Minimize interruptions.

Note. DO NOT remove the heel of your hand from the casualty's chest or reposition your hands between compressions.

15-5. Open the airway. See Chapter 3, Task 081-COM-1023, on page 3-1.

Note. There are two methods to opening of the airway to provide breaths, the head-tilt chin-lift or the jaw thrust.

15-6. Give two full rescue breaths.

- Move quickly to the casualty's head and lean over his mouth.
- Give two full rescue breaths (each lasting 1 second).

Note. Deliver air over one second to make the casualty's chest rise.

15-7. Continue to alternate between chest compressions and ventilations (30:2) until—

- The casualty is revived.
- You are too exhausted to continue.
- You are relieved by a health care provider.
- The casualty is pronounced dead by an authorized person.
- A second rescuer states, *I know CPR*, and joins you in performing two-rescuer CPR.

15-8. Limit pulse checks.

15-9. Perform two-rescuer CPR, if applicable, as follows:

Note. When performing two-rescuer CPR, the rescuers must change position every 2 minutes to avoid fatigue and increase the effectiveness of compressions.

- Compressor—
  - Give 30 chest compressions at the rate of 100 per minute.
  - Compress the chest at least 2 inches (5 centimeters).
  - Allow the chest to recoil completely after each compression.
  - Minimize interruptions in compressions, (limit any interruptions to less than 10 seconds).
  - Count compressions aloud.

- Switch duties with the second rescuer every 5 cycles or about 2 minutes, taking less than 5 seconds to switch.

- Ventilator—
  - Maintain an open airway. See Chapter 3, Task 081-COM-1023, on page 3-1.

CAUTION

DO NOT push on the abdomen. If the casualty vomits, turn the casualty on his side, clear the airway (suction if available, usually provided by medical personnel/units), and continue CPR (if you suspect trauma, logroll the casualty as a unit), clear the airway, and then continue CPR.

- Give breaths, watching for chest rise and avoiding excessive ventilation.

Note. If signs of gastric distention are noted, do the following: 1. Recheck and reposition the airway. 2. Watch for the rise and fall of the chest. 3. Ventilate the casualty only enough to cause the chest to rise.

- Encourage the first rescuer/compressor to perform compressions that are deep enough and fast enough to allow complete chest recoil between compressions.
- Continue CPR switching duties as described in paragraph 15-8.

Note. The rescuer doing rescue breathing should recheck the carotid pulse every 3 to 5 minutes.

CAUTION

During evacuation, CPR or rescue breathing should be continued en route if necessary.

15-10. Continue evaluating the casualty when the pulse and breathing are restored. If the casualty's condition permits, place him in the recovery position. See Chapter 3, Task 081-COM 1023, on page 3-1.

15-11. Seek medical aid.

15-12. Document the procedure on the TCCC Card (DD Form 1380).

This page intentionally left blank.

Chapter 16
Head Injuries (081-833-0038)

TYPES OF HEAD INJURIES

16-1 Head injuries range from minor abrasions or cuts to severe brain injuries that may result in unconsciousness and death. Head injuries are classified as open or closed. An open head injury is visible and has evidence of bleeding. A closed head injury may be visible (such as a depression in the skull), or the wound may not be visible (such as internal bleeding) and not visibly apparent. Some head injuries may cause unconsciousness; however, some very serious head injuries may not result in unconsciousness. Casualties with head and neck injuries should be treated as though they also may have a spinal injury. The casualty should not be moved until the head and neck are stabilized unless he is in immediate danger (such as close to a burning vehicle). Prompt first aid measures should be initiated for casualties with suspected head injuries. **Always seek medical aid for any type of head injury.**

CLOSED HEAD INJURIES

WARNING

Brain injury, leading to a loss of function or death, often occurs without evidence of a skull fracture or scalp injury. Because the skull cannot expand, swelling of the brain or a collection of fluid pressing on the brain can cause pressure. This can compress and destroy brain tissue.

16-2 A closed head injury caused by a direct blow to the head can result in—

- Deformity to the head.
- Clear fluid or blood escaping from the nose and/or ear(s).
- Periorbital discoloration (raccoon eyes).
- Bruising behind the ears, over the mastoid process (battle sign).
- Lowered pulse rate if the casualty has not lost a significant amount of blood.

16-3 Signs of increased intracranial (inside the skull) pressure include—

- Headache, nausea, and/or vomiting.
- Possible unconsciousness.
- Change in pupil size and symmetry (equal/same size).
- Lateral loss of motor nerve function-one side of the body becomes paralyzed.

Note. Lateral loss may not happen immediately but may occur later.

- Change in the casualty's respiratory rate or pattern.
- Elevated body temperature.
- Restlessness (indicates insufficient oxygenation of the brain).

CONCUSSION

16-4 A concussion is caused by a violent jar or shock and can result in—

- Temporary unconsciousness followed by confusion.
- Temporary, usually short term, loss of some or all brain functions.
- The casualty has a headache or is seeing double.
- The casualty may or may not have a skull fracture.

Note. A direct blow to the skull may bruise the brain.

CONTUSION

16-5 A contusion is an internal bruise or injury. It is more serious than a concussion. A contusion may result in—

- The injured tissue may bleed or swell.
- Swelling may cause increased intracranial (inside the skull) pressure that may result in decreased level of consciousness and even death.

OPEN HEAD INJURY

16-6 An open head injury is notable for blood loss from the very vascular nature of the head and neck area. An open head injury may result in—

- Penetrating wound-an entry wound with no exit wound.
- Perforating wound-the wound has both entry and exit wounds.
- Visibly deformed skull.
- Exposed brain tissue.
- Possible unconsciousness.
- Paralysis or disability on one side of the body.
- Change in pupil size.
- Lacerated scalp tissue-may have extensive bleeding.

FIRST AID FOR HEAD INJURIES

16-7 Provide direct manual stabilization of the head as follows:

- Place your hands on each side of the casualty's head, thereby, maintaining the position of the head in line with the body.
- Support, or have someone support the head in this fashion.

16-8 Assess the casualty's level of consciousness by the following method:

- Alert, Voice, Pain, Unconscious Method.
- Is the casualty alert?
- Does the casualty respond to verbal stimuli/commands?
- Does the casualty respond to painful stimulus?
- Is the casualty unconscious?

INITIATE TREATMENT FOR A SUPERFICIAL HEAD INJURY

16-9 Provide first aid for superficial head injury as follows:

- Apply a dressing.
- Observe for abnormal behavior or evidence of complications.

HEAD INJURY INVOLVING TRAUMA

16-10 Provide first aid for head injury involving trauma as follows:

- Maintain a patent airway using the jaw thrust maneuver.
- Dress the head wounds.

> **WARNING**
>
> **DO NOT apply pressure to or replace brain tissue.**

- Control bleeding.
- Treat for shock.
- Seek medical aid.
- Monitor the casualty for convulsions or seizures.

> **CAUTION**
>
> DO NOT give the casualty anything by mouth.

16-11 Monitor unstable casualties for the following—

- Level of consciousness by using the before described; alert, responds to voice, reacts to pain stimuli, and is the casualty unconscious indicators. Is the casualty aware and alert?
- Pupils respond to light and are equal in size.
- Motor functions, casualty's strength, mobility, coordination and sensation.
- Seek medical aid.
- Evacuate the casualty as soon as possible.

This page intentionally left blank.

Chapter 17

Abdominal Injuries (081-831-0028)

17-1. The most serious abdominal wound is one which an object penetrates the abdominal wall and pierces internal organs or large blood vessels. In these instances, bleeding may be severe and death can occur rapidly.

17-2. Position the casualty as follows:

- Place the casualty on his back (face up).
- Flex the casualty's knees.
- Turn the casualty's head to the side and keep the airway clear if vomiting occurs.

> **WARNING**
>
> **The most important concern in the initial first aid of abdominal injuries is shock. Shock may be present initially or develop later. Neither the presence nor absence of a wound, nor the size of the external wound is a safe guideline for judging the severity of the wound.**

- Initiate treatment for shock. See Chapter 8, Task 081-COM-1005, on page 8-1.

> **CAUTION**
>
> DO NOT attempt to replace protruding internal organs or remove any protruding foreign objects.

- Expose the wound. Inspect for distention, contusions, penetration, eviscerations or obvious bleeding.
- It may be necessary to use improvised dressings (if there are two wounds, entry and exit) for example strips of cloth, a T-shirt, or the cleanest material available.

17-3. Stabilize any protruding objects. See Chapter 18, Task 081-833-0029, on page 18-1.

17-4. Apply a sterile abdominal dressing as follows:

Note. Protruding abdominal organs should be kept moist to prevent the tissue from drying out. A moist sterile dressing should be applied if available.

- Using the sterile side of the dressing, or other clean material, place any protruding organs near the wound. (DO NOT try to push organs back inside the body.)
- Ensure that the dressing is large enough to cover the entire mass of protruding organs or area of the wound.
- If large enough to cover the affected area, place the sterile side of the plastic wrapper directly over the wound.
- Place the dressing directly on top of the wound or plastic wrapper, if used.

CAUTION

DO NOT apply pressure on the wound or expose internal parts/organs.

- Tie the dressings loosely at the casualty's side.

17-5. If two dressings are needed to cover a large wound, repeat steps in paragraph 17-2. If necessary, loosely cover the dressing with cravats. Tie them on the side of the casualty opposite to that of the dressing ties.

17-6. To avoid causing further injury to the casualty—

- Do not touch any exposed organs.
- Do not try to push any exposed organs back into the body.
- Do not tie the dressing tails tightly or directly over the wound.
- Do not give the casualty anything by mouth.

Note. Continue to evaluate the casualty and provide necessary first aid.

17-7. Prepare the casualty for evacuation as follows:

- Place the casualty on his back (face up) with the knees flexed.
- If evacuation is delayed, check the casualty for shock every 5 minutes.
- Seek medical aid.
- Record the procedures applied on the TCCC Card (DD Form 1380).

Chapter 18

Impalement Injuries (081-833-0029)

18-1. Dependent upon where the impaled object is located on the body, extreme care must be exercised. Improper methods may cause severe injury and possess the potential for further disability and death.

WARNING

DO NOT exert any force on or attempt to remove the impaled object unless the object is impaled in the cheek and both ends of the object can be seen or unless the object is blocking the airway. Severe bleeding or nerve and muscle damage may result.

18-2. Apply first aid for an impaled object as follows:

- Tell the casualty to remain still and not to move the impaled object.
- Expose the injury by cutting away or removing clothing or equipment around the wound site.
- If the impalement is on an extremity, check the pulse distal (situated away from the center of the body or injury) from the injury site.
- If the impalement is found in the cheek and both ends of the object can be seen, perform the following:
  - Remove the object in the direction it entered the cheek.
  - Position the casualty to allow for drainage.
  - If both ends of the object in the cheek cannot be seen, immobilize the impaled object.

Note. If an assistant is available, one person should immobilize the object while the other applies the dressings and bandages.

WARNING

DO NOT exert force on the object.

- If necessary, apply direct pressure using gloved hands on either side of the object.
- Place several layers of bulky dressings around the injury site so that the dressings surround the object.
- Use additional bulky materials or dressings to build up the area around the object.
- Apply the support bandages.
- Apply the bandage over the bulky support material to hold it in place.

WARNING

DO NOT anchor the bandage on or exert pressure on the impaled object.

- Apply the bandage tightly but not so tightly as to impair circulation or breathing.
- Check circulation after applying the support bandages.

Note. If a pulse was palpated (felt) on an extremity and cannot be palpated after the bandage has been applied, the bandage must be loosened until a pulse can be palpated.

WARNING

Do NOT anchor a splint or sling to the impaled object. Avoid undue motion of the impaled object when applying a splint.

- Immobilize the affected area with a splint or sling, if applicable.
- Check for a pulse distal (far side of the wound) to the injury site.
- Treat for shock, if necessary.
- Seek medical assistance.

Chapter 19

Apply an Elastic Bandage (081-933-0264)

19-1. Select the appropriate bandage material for the injury as follows:

Note. The width of the bandage to use is determined by the size of the part to be covered. As a general rule; the larger the part or the area, the wider the bandage applied.

- Use gauze or a gauze bandage roll for bleeding injuries of the hand, wrist, elbow, shoulder, groin, knee, ankle, and foot.
- Use an elastic roller bandage for amputations, arterial bleeding, sprains, and torn muscles as follows:
  - Hand: 2-inch bandage.
  - Lower arm, lower leg, and foot: 3-inch bandage.
  - Thigh and chest: 4- to 6-inch bandage.

Note. Elastic roller bandages may be used whenever pressure support or restriction of movement is needed. They should not be used to secure dressings.

19-1. Prepare the patient for bandaging as follows:

- Position the body part to be bandaged in a normal resting position (position of function).

Note. Bending a bandaged joint changes the pressure of the bandage in places of stress (elbow, knee, and ankle).

- Ensure the body part to be bandaged is clean and dry.
- Place pads over bony places or between skin surfaces to be bandaged (such as fingers and armpits).

CAUTION

DO NOT wrap too tightly. The roller bandage may act as a tourniquet on an injured limb, causing further damage.

19-1. Apply the anchor wrap by—

- Laying the bandage end at an angle across the area to be bandaged.
- Bringing the bandage under the area, back to the starting point, and make a second turn.
- Folding the uncovered triangle of the bandage end back over the second turn.
- Covering the triangle with a third turn, completing the anchor.

19-1. Apply the bandage wrap to the injury as follows:

- Use a circular wrap to end other bandage patterns, such as a pressure bandage, or to cover small dressings.
- Use a spiral wrap for a large cylindrical area such as a forearm, upper arm, calf, or thigh. The spiral wrap is used to cover an area larger than a circular wrap can cover.
- Use a reverse spiral wrap to cover small to large conical areas, for the example, from ankle to knee.

- Use a figure eight wrap to support or limit joint movement at the hand, elbow, knee, ankle, or foot.
- Use a spica wrap (same as the figure eight wrap) to cover a much larger area such as the hip or shoulder.
- Use a recurrent wrap for anchoring a dressing on fingers, the head, or on a stump.

Note. Bandage width depends on the site, 1-inch wide for fingers and 3-, 4-, or 6-inches wide for the stump or head.

19-1. Check circulation after application of the bandage as follows:
- Check the pulse distal (away from the anatomical center) to the injury.
- Check for capillary refill (under the fingernails or toenails) less than 2 seconds is normal, if applicable.
- Inspect the skin below the bandaging for discoloration.
- Ask the patient if any numbness, coldness, or tingling sensations are felt in the bandaged part.
- Remove and reapply the bandage, if necessary.

19-1. Check for irritation as follows:
- Ask the casualty if the bandage rubs.
- Check the bandage for wrinkles near the skin surface.
- Check for red skin or sores (ulcers) when the bandage is removed.
- Remove and reapply the bandage, if necessary.

19-1. Elevate injured extremities to reduce swelling (edema) and control bleeding, if appropriate.

19-1. Record the procedures on TCCC Card (DD Form 1380).

19-1. Seek medical aid.

19-10. Evacuate the casualty if necessary.

Chapter 20

Apply a Sling and Swath (081-833-0265)

20-1. A sling is a triangular bandage used to support the shoulder and arm. Once the casualty's arm is placed in a sling, a swath can be used to hold the arm against the side of the chest. To apply a sling—

- Evaluate distal circulation (for example, the radial pulse [at the wrist]; the posterior tibial pulse [on the inside of the ankle]), sensation, and motor functions of the extremity.
- Prepare the sling by folding cloth into a triangle.

Note. A triangular bandage makes an ideal arm sling.

- Fold the injured arm across the casualty's chest.

Note. If the casualty cannot hold their arm, have someone assist them until you tie the sling.

- Position the sling over the top of the casualty's chest.
- Extend one point of the triangle beyond the elbow on the injured side.
- Take the bottom point and bring it up over the casualty's arm.
- Continue to take it over the top of the injured shoulder.
- If appropriate, draw up the ends of the sling so that the casualty's hand is about 4 inches above the elbow.

CAUTION

If a spinal injury is suspected, do not tie the sling around the casualty's neck, instead, pin the ends to the casualty's clothing securely.

- Tie the ends of the sling together.
- Make sure the knot does not press against the back of the casualty's neck.
- Pad with bulky dressings.
- Confirm the casualty's fingertips are left exposed.
- Evaluate circulation, sensation, and motor function.
- If pulse has been lost, take off the sling and repeat the procedure.
- If procedure was repeated, recheck circulation, sensation, and motor function.
- Form a pocket for the casualty's elbow.
- Take hold of the point of material at the elbow and fold it forward, pinning it to the front of the sling.
- If you do not have a pin, twist the excess material and tie a knot in the point.

20-2. To hold the sling securely next to the body, apply a swath as follows:

- Form a swath from a second piece of material by tying it around the chest and the injured arm, over the sling.

Note. Do not place it over the casualty's arm on the uninjured side.

- Reevaluate circulation, sensation, and motor function.
- Monitor casualty until evacuation.

This page intentionally left blank.

Chapter 21

Treat a Casualty for Snakebite (081-833-0073)

21-1. When encountering a casualty with snakebite, scan the ground around the area to ensure the scene is safe. Stay calm and take necessary body substance isolation precautions.

21-1. Expose the injury site.

> **WARNING**
>
> **Each person reacts differently to a snakebite. You should consider the bite from any known poisonous snake or any unidentified snake, to be an emergency.**

> **CAUTION**
>
> If the bite cannot be positively identified as nonpoisonous, the bite should be treated as a poisonous bite. Do not delay treatment during this step.

21-1. Determine the type of snakebite as follows:

Note. Staying calm and keeping the casualty calm and at rest is critical.

- Nonpoisonous—
  - Four to six rows of teeth.
  - No fangs.
- Poisonous—
  - Two rows of teeth.
  - Two fangs which create puncture wounds.

> **WARNING**
>
> **Exception is the coral snake, a poisonous snake that does not have fangs. It leaves a semicircular pattern with its teeth as it *chews* the skin.**

  - Elliptical pupils or vertical slits, much like those of a cat.
  - Pit between the eye and mouth.
  - A variety of different-shaped blotches on backgrounds of pink, yellow, olive, tan, gray, or brown skin.

Note. The exception to color is the coral snake which is ringed with red, yellow and black. An old ditty is offered to assist in identifying a coral snake, *red on yellow will kill a fellow, red on black, venom it will lack.*

21-1. Check the casualty for the following signs and symptoms of a poisonous snakebite:

Note. The signs and symptoms of a poisonous snakebite generally occur immediately.

- A noticeable bite on the skin which may appear as nothing more than discoloration.
- Pain and swelling in the area of the bite, which may be slow to develop, taking from 30 minutes to several hours.
- Rapid pulse and labored breathing.
- Progressive general weakness.
- Vision problems (dim or blurred).
- Seizures.
- Shock.
- Dizziness or faintness.
- Fever, chills, or sweating.
- Nausea and vomiting.
- Drowsiness or unconsciousness.
- Paralysis.
- Coma.

WARNING

Never delay care and transport in order to capture the snake.

CAUTION

Do not give the casualty any sedatives, alcohol, food, or tobacco.

21-1. Initiate treatment as follows:

Note. If the dead or captured snake is at the scene, it is not your role to identify the snake, but to place it in a sealed container and transport it along with the casualty.

- Never scrub the area or apply a cold pack to snakebites. There may only one fang mark.
- For nonpoisonous snakebite—
  - Wash the area around the bite gently using mild or a strong soap solution and sterile saline (if available), or clean water.
  - If the casualty has a current tetanus toxoid series, refer, transport the casualty to the medical officer or doctor.
  - If the casualty does not have a current tetanus toxoid series, transport the casualty to a medical treatment facility.

- For poisonous snakebite—

> **WARNING**
>
> **DO NOT cut the bite and suction or squeeze the bite site.**

  - Wash the area around the bite gently using a mild or strong soap and sterile normal saline if available, otherwise, clean water.
  - Keep the casualty calm and reassured.
  - Explain to the casualty what will be done.
  - Limit their physical activity.
  - Keep any bitten extremities immobilized-the application of a splint will help.
  - Lower the injection site below the level of the heart.
  - Remove any rings, bracelets, or other constricting items on the bitten extremity.

Note. Removing jewelry or other constricting objects from the casualty's affected limb will help in case the limb swells, which could make removal more difficult later.

- Seek medical assistance and direction as follows:
  - Ask for the best receiving medical facility where antivenom is most readily available to treat the casualty.
  - Ask medical direction and follow local protocols or instructions in the application of a constricting band in the first aid of snakebite, proximal to the bite.
  - Record first aid applied on the TCCC Card (DD Form 1380).
- Evacuate the casualty.

Note. Rapid transport and administration of antivenom are the most effective interventions for the treatment of life-threatening snakebites.

21-1. If accompanying the casualty on CASEVAC to a medical treatment facility, observe the casualty carefully for signs and symptoms of allergic reaction, monitoring the airway, breathing, circulation, vital signs (for first aid purposes; pulse and respiration), distal pulse of the bitten extremity, treating for shock, and conserving body heat.

This page intentionally left blank.

Chapter 22

Initiate Treatment for Anaphylactic Shock (081-833-0003)

22-1. When initiating first aid for anaphylactic shock it is imperative **to seek medical assistance immediately** and acquire the casualty's epinephrine autoinjector if available.

Note. Anaphylactic reactions occur within minutes or even seconds after contact with the substance to which the casualty is allergic. Reactions occur in the skin, respiratory system, and circulatory system.

22-1. Check the casualty for signs and symptoms of anaphylactic shock as follows:

- Skin—
  - Flushed or ashen.
  - Burning or itching.
  - Edema (swelling), especially in the face, tongue, or airway.
  - Urticaria (hives) spreading over the body.
  - Marked swelling of the lips and cyanosis about the lips.
- Respiratory—
  - Tightness in or pain in the chest.
  - Sneezing and coughing.
  - Wheezing, stridor (high pitched wheezing sound) or difficulty in breathing (dyspnea).
  - Sputum (may be blood tinged).
  - Respiratory failure.
- Circulatory—
  - Weak, rapid pulse.
  - Falling blood pressure.
  - Hypotension.
  - Dizziness or fainting.
  - Coma.
- Open the airway, if necessary. See Chapter 3, Task 081-COM-1023, on page 3-1.
- Seek medical assistance and transportation immediately concurrent with providing first aid measures. Send a runner or have a bystander call for help.

Note. In cases of airway obstruction from swelling of the airway, trained medical intervention is required.

- Administer the casualty's autoinjector, if available, as follows:
  - Pediatric autoinjector single dose, 0.15 milligrams, adult autoinjector single dose for greater than 66 pounds, 0.3 milligrams. Follow the directions for administration and use provided with the autoinjector.

Note. Annotate the time of injection on the TCCC Card (DD Form 1380).

  - Additional epinephrine may be required if anaphylaxis progresses. Additional dose may be administered every 5 to 10 minutes if the casualty has been prescribed additional autoinjectors.

- Provide supportive measures for the treatment of shock, respiratory failure, circulatory collapse, or cardiac arrest as follows:
  - Position the casualty in the supine position (on his back) with legs elevated if injuries permit.
  - Perform rescue breathing, if necessary. See Chapter 14, Task 081-831-0048, on page 14-1.
  - Administer external chest compressions, if necessary. See Chapter 15, Task 081-831-0046, on page 15-1.
- Check the casualty's vital signs (pulse and respiration) every 3 to 5 minutes until the casualty is stable.
- Record the first aid provided on the TCCC Card (DD Form 1380).
- Request medical evacuation for the casualty. The use of CASEVAC is not recommended, with the exception, if no medical evacuation is available. The casualty must be taken to the nearest medical treatment facility as soon as possible.

Chapter 23

Transport a Casualty (081-COM-1046)

23-1. Transporting a casualty away from danger or to an evacuation vehicle is a key component of first aid. Care must be exercised in order not to further injure the casualty. More information concerning the transport and evacuation of casualties is found in STP 8-68W13-SM-TG and in ATPs 4-25.13 and 4-02.2. The movement of casualties requires risk assessment. See ATP 5-19 for more information.

> **WARNING**
>
> **If the casualty was involved in a vehicle crash you should always consider that he may have a spinal injury. Unless there is an immediate life-threatening situation (such as fire, explosion), DO NOT move the casualty with a suspected back or neck injury. Seek medical personnel for guidance on how to transport the casualty.**

REMOVING A CASUALTY FROM A VEHICLE

23-2. To remove a casualty from a vehicle if necessary, laterally—

- With the assistance of another Soldier, grasp the casualty's arms and legs.
- While stabilizing the casualty's head and neck as much as possible, lift the casualty free of the vehicle and move him to a safe place on the ground.

Note. If medical personnel are available, they may stabilize the casualty's head, neck, and upper body with a special board or splint.

23-3. To remove a casualty from a vehicle if necessary, upward—

Note. You may have to remove a casualty upward from a vehicle; for example, from the passenger compartment of a wheeled vehicle lying on its side, or from the hatch of an armored vehicle sitting upright.

- You may place a pistol belt or similar material around the casualty's chest to help pull him from the vehicle.
- With the assistance of another Soldier inside the vehicle, draw the casualty upward using the pistol belt or similar material or by grasping his arms.
- While stabilizing the casualty's head and neck as much as possible, lift the casualty free of the vehicle and place him on the topmost side of the vehicle.

Note. If medical personnel are available, they may stabilize the casualty's head, neck, and upper body with a special board or splint.

- Depending on the situation, move the casualty from the topmost side of the vehicle to a safe place on the ground.

WARNING

DO NOT use manual carries to move a casualty with a neck or spine injury, unless a life-threatening hazard is in the immediate area. Seek medical guidance on how to move and transport the casualty.

TYPES OF MANUAL CARRIES

23-4. Manual carries are used to move a casualty a short distance to a safer location (cover), a greater level of care, or to a medical evacuation vehicle or a CASEVAC transport.

23-5. Select an appropriate method to transport the casualty as follows:

Note. The fireman's carry is the typical one-man carry practiced in training. However, in reality, with a fully equipped casualty, it is nearly impossible to lift a Soldier over your shoulder and move to cover quickly.

- Fireman's carry—use for an unconscious or severely injured casualty.

CAUTION

DO NOT use the neck drag if the casualty has a broken arm or a suspected neck injury.

- Neck drag—use in combat for short distances.
- Cradle-drop drag—use to move a casualty who cannot walk when being moved up or down stairs.
- Use litters if materials are available, if the casualty must be moved a long distance, or if manual carries will cause further injury.

EVACUATE THE CASUALTY USING THE APPROPRIATE TYPE OF CARRY

23-6. Once the appropriate type of carry is selected, evacuate the casualty.

23-7. Conduct a Fireman's carry by using the following procedures:

- Kneel at the casualty's uninjured side.
- Place the casualty's arms above his head.
- Cross the ankle on the uninjured side over the opposite ankle.
- Place one of your hands on the shoulder farther from you and your other hand on his hip or thigh.
- Roll the casualty toward you onto his abdomen.
- Straddle the casualty.

Note. Care must be taken to keep the casualty's head from falling backward, resulting in a neck injury.

- Place your hands under the casualty's chest and lock them together.
- Lift the casualty to his knees as you move backward.

- Continue to move backwards, thus straightening the casualty's legs and locking the knees.
- Walk forward, bringing the casualty to a standing position but tilted slightly backward to prevent the knees from buckling.
- Maintain constant support of the casualty with one arm. Free your other arm, quickly grasp his wrist, and raise the arm high.
- Quickly pass your head under the casualty's raised arm, releasing it as you pass under it.
- Move swiftly to face the casualty.
- Secure your arms around his waist.
- Immediately place your foot between his feet and spread them (approximately 6 to 8 inches apart).
- Again grasp the casualty's wrist and raise the arm high above your head.
- Bend down and pull the casualty's arm over and down your shoulder bringing his body across your shoulders. At the same time pass your arm between the legs.
- Grasp the casualty's wrist with one hand while placing your other hand on your knee for support.
- Rise with the casualty correctly positioned.

Note. Your other hand is free to use as needed.

WARNING

DO NOT use the neck drag if the casualty has a fractured arm or a suspected neck injury. If the casualty is unconscious, protect his head from the ground.

23-8. Conduct a neck drag by using the following procedures:

- Place the casualty on his back, if not already there, otherwise, use the following steps:
  - Kneel at the casualty's uninjured side.
  - Place the casualty's arm above his head.
  - Cross the ankle on the injured side over the opposite ankle.
  - Place one of your hands on the shoulder farther from you and your other hand on his hip or thigh.
  - Roll the casualty toward you onto his abdomen.
- Once the casualty is on his back, tie the casualty's hands at the wrists. (If conscious, the casualty may clasp his hands together around your neck.)
- Straddle the casualty in a kneeling face-to-face position.
- Loop the casualty's tied hands over and around your neck.
- Crawl forward, looking ahead, dragging the casualty with you.

23-9. Conduct a cradle drop drag by using the following procedures:

- With the casualty lying on his back, kneel at the head.
- Slide your hands, palms up, under the casualty's shoulders.
- Get a firm hold under his armpits.
- Partially rise, supporting the casualty's head on one of your forearms.

Note. You may bring your elbows together and let the casualty's head rest on both of your forearms.

- With the casualty in a semi-sitting position, rise and drag the casualty backwards.
- Back down the steps (or up if appropriate), supporting the casualty's head and body and letting the hips and legs drop from step to step.

LITTERS

23-10. When possible, a casualty should be transported on a litter rather than using a manual carry. A litter has many advantages as delineated in ATP 4-25.13.

POLYMER FLEXIBLE LITTER

23-11. Evacuate the casualty using a commercial polymer flexible litter (referred further in the text as a flexible litter, or litter). First prepare the flexible litter for transport by—

- Removing the flexible litter from the pack and placing it on the ground.
- Unfastening the retainer strap.
- Stepping on the foot end of the flexible litter and unrolling the flexible litter completely.
- Bending the flexible litter in half and back roll.
- Repeating with the opposite end of the litter so that the flexible litter lays flat.
- Pointing out the handholds, straps for the casualty, and dragline at the head of the litter.

23-12. Place and secure a casualty onto to a flexible litter by conducting the following:

- Place the flexible litter next to the casualty so that the head end of the litter is next to the casualty's head.
- Place the cross straps under the flexible litter.
- Log roll the casualty onto his side in a steady and even manner.
- Slide the flexible litter as far under the casualty as possible.
- Gently roll the casualty until he is again lying on his back with the litter beneath him.
- Slide the casualty to the middle of the flexible litter, keeping his spinal column as straight as possible.
- Pull out the strap from under the flexible litter.
- Bring the straps across the casualty.
- Lift the sides of the flexible litter and fasten the four cross straps to the buckles directly opposite the straps.
- Lift the foot portion of the flexible litter.
- Feed the foot straps over the casualty's lower extremities and through the unused grommets at the foot end of the flexible litter.

23-13. Lift the casualty by—

Note. For a flexible litter, lift the sides of the flexible litter and fasten the four cross straps to the buckles directly opposite the straps. Lift the foot portion of the flexible litter and feed the foot straps through the unused grommets at the foot end of the flexible litter and fasten the buckles.

- Using for Soldiers (two on each side), all facing the casualty's feet. Have each Soldier grab a handle with their inside hand.
- In one fluid motion on the preparatory command of *prepare to lift* and then command of execution of *lift*, raise as a unit holding the casualty parallel and even.

MULTIHINGED FOLDING LITTER

23-14. A multihinged folding litter (referred further in the text as a multihinged litter, or litter), is often used in tactical situations where compact size is valued. When unfolded, the litter approximates the dimensions of a standard litter.

23-15. Evacuate a casualty by preparing a multihinged litter for use by—

- Removing the litter from the bag.
- Standing the litter upright and releasing buckles from the litter.
- Placing the litter on the ground and completely extending it with the fabric side facing up.
- Keeping the multihinged litter as straight as possible, grab the handles and rotate them inwards until all the hinges rotate and lock.

Note. This action is done best by using two individuals on each end of the litter executing this step simultaneously.

- While maintaining the hinges in the locked position, apply firm, steady pressure on the spreader bar with your foot. Increase pressure with your foot until the spreader bar locks into place.

23-16. Place the casualty on the litter as follows:

- Place the litter next to the casualty. Ensure that the head end of the litter is beside the head of the casualty.
- Log roll the casualty and slide the litter as far under him as possible. Gently roll the casualty down onto the litter.
- Slide the casualty to the center of the litter. Be sure to keep the spinal column as straight as possible.
- Secure the casualty to the litter using litter straps or other available materials.

IMPROVISED LITTERS

23-17. There are times when a casualty may have to be moved and a standard litter is not available. Evacuate a casualty by using an improvised litter. More improvised litters are found in ATP 4-25.13.

Poncho Improvised Litter

23-18. Use a poncho with two poles or limbs as follows:

- Open the poncho and lay the two poles lengthwise across the center forming three equal sections.
- Reach in, pull the hood up toward you, and lay it flat on the poncho.
- Fold on section of the poncho over the first pole.
- Fold the remaining section of the poncho over the second pole to the first pole.

Jacket Improvised Litter

23-19. Use shirts or jackets and two poles or limbs by using the following procedure:

- Zipper closed two uniform jackets and turn them inside out, leaving the sleeves inside.
- Lay the jackets on the ground and pass through the sleeves, leaving one at the top and one at the bottom of the poles to support the casualty's whole body.

23-20. Place the casualty on the improvised litter by using the following procedure:

- Lift the litter.
- Place the litter next to the casualty. Ensure the head end of the litter is adjacent to the head of the casualty.
- Slide the casualty to the center of the litter. Be sure to keep the spinal column as straight as possible.
- Secure the casualty to the litter using litter straps or other available materials.

Load Casualties onto a Military Vehicle

23-21. Information concerning ground ambulances, air ambulances, and CASEVAC is found in ATP 4-02.2 and STP 8-68W13-SM-TG.

Ground Ambulance

Note. Ground ambulances have combat medics to take care of the casualties during evacuation. Follow any special instructions they give for loading, securing, or unloading casualties.

23-22. When loading a ground ambulance, use the following procedures:

- Make sure each litter casualty is secured to his litter. Use the litter straps when available.
- Load the most serious casualty last.
- Load the casualty head first (head in the direction of travel) rather than feet first.
- Make sure each litter is secured to the vehicle.

Note. Unload casualties in reverse order, most seriously injured casualty first.

Air Ambulance

Note. Air ambulances have combat medics (flight medics) to take care of the casualties during evacuation. Follow any special instructions that they give for loading, securing, or unloading casualties.

23-23. When loading air ambulances, use the following procedures and precautions:

- Remain 50 yards from the helicopter until the litter squad is signaled to approach the aircraft.

WARNING

Never go around the rear of the UH-60 or UH-1 aircraft.

- Approach the aircraft in full view of the aircraft crew, maintaining visual confirmation that the crew is aware of the approach of the litter party. Ensure that the aircrew can continue to visually distinguish friendly from enemy personnel at all times. Maintain a low silhouette when approaching the aircraft.
- Approach UH-60 and UH-1 aircraft from the sides. Do not approach from front or rear. If you must move to the opposite side of the aircraft, approach from the side the exterior of the aircraft. Then hug the skin of the aircraft, and move around the front of the aircraft to the other side.
- Approach CH-47 aircraft from the rear.
- Approach MH-53 aircraft from the sides to the rear ramp, avoiding the tail rotor.
- Approach nonstandard aircraft in full view of the crew, avoiding tail rotors, main rotors, propellers, and jet intakes.

- Approach performance aircraft (M/C-130, C-17, and C-5B) from the rear, under the guidance of the aircraft loadmaster or the ground control party.
- Load the most seriously injured casualty last.
- Load the casualty who will occupy the upper berth first, and then load the next litter casualty immediately under the first casualty.

Note. This is done to keep the casualty from accidentally falling on another casualty if his litter is dropped before it is secured.

- When casualties are placed lengthwise, position them with their heads toward the direction of travel.
- Make sure each litter casualty is secured to the litter.
- Make sure each litter is secured to the aircraft.

Note. Unload casualties in reverse order, most seriously injured first.

Ground Military Vehicles

23-24. Ground military vehicles used to transport casualties are referred to as CASEVAC. When nonmedical military vehicles are used, medical equipment and oftentimes medical personnel are not present. See FM 4-02, ATPs 4-02.2 and 4-02.3 for information and appropriate cautions when using CASEVAC for transport of casualties.

Note 1. Nonmedical military vehicles may be used to evacuate casualties when no medical evacuation vehicles are available.

Note 2. If medical personnel are present, follow their instructions for loading, securing, and unloading casualties.

23-25. The following are guidelines for loading casualties into a ground evacuation vehicle:

- When loading casualties into the vehicle, load the most seriously injured last.
- When the casualty is loaded lengthwise, load the casualty with his head pointing forward, toward the direction of travel.
- Ensure each casualty is secured to the litter. Use litter straps if available.
- Secure each litter to the vehicle as it is loaded into place. Make sure each litter is secured.

Note. Unload casualties in reverse order, most seriously injured casualty first.

This page intentionally left blank.

★Chapter 24

Initiate First Aid for Lacerations of the Eyelid (081-833-0040) With IFAK Eye-Shield

SURVEY

24-1. Survey the situation, if the injury is from chemical exposure, immediately wash the eye (see Task 081-833-0044). Otherwise, DO NOT put anything on the eye ITSELF, especially if you think the eye is cut.

24-2. If necessary, remove the casualty's headgear. Position and treat the casualty as follows:

- Conscious casualty will be placed in a seated position.
- Unconscious casualty will be placed in a supine position with the head slightly elevated.
- Gently clean any dirt or blood from the affected area around the eye.

> **WARNING**
>
> **DO NOT put pressure on the eye or remove anything from the eye surface. This could cause additional harm, such as loss of eyesight or loss of the eye.**

24-3. Examine the eyes for the following:

- Objects protruding from the eyes.
- Look for foreign objects in or on eyes and damage to the eyes.
- Swelling or lacerations of the eyes.
- Bloodshot appearance of the white of the eyes.
- Bleeding—
  - Surrounding the eye.
  - From inside the eyeball.
  - Coming from the eyeball.

24-4. Ask the casualty if he is wearing contact lenses, but DO NOT force the eyelids open. Record and communicate to medical personnel (first responders, emergency medical technicians, or combat medics) that contact lenses are being worn.

24-5. Categorize the injury as follows:

- Injury to the tissue surrounding the eye (lacerations and contusions).
- Injury to the eyeball. (See Task 081-833-0039.)
- Extrusion (the eye is protruding out of the eye socket). (See Task 081-833-0042.)
- Foreign bodies. (See Task 081-833-0039.)
- Protruding (impaled) objects. (See Task 081-833-0039.)

SHIELD

24-6. Provide first aid for the injury as follows:

Note. Torn eyelids should be handled carefully. Wrap any fragments in a separate moist dressing and evacuate with the casualty.

- Control bleeding with light pressure from a dressing.
- Gently clean any dirt or blood from the affected area around the eye.

WARNING

DO NOT use any pressure if you suspect that the eyeball itself has been injured.

- Cover the eyelid with the rigid eye-shield provided in the IFAK, the joint first aid kit, or anything that provides a hard cover over the eye such as—
  - Eye protective gear—ballistic glasses or goggles.
  - The bottom of a disposable cup, for example one made of extruded polystyrene (foam), plastic, or paper.

Note. This helps prevent any undue pressure or further damage to the eye.

  - Secure the shield by applying tape from the cheek to the forehead (see Figure 24-1). If no tape is available, use gauze, cloth dressing, shoelace, or string to secure in place.

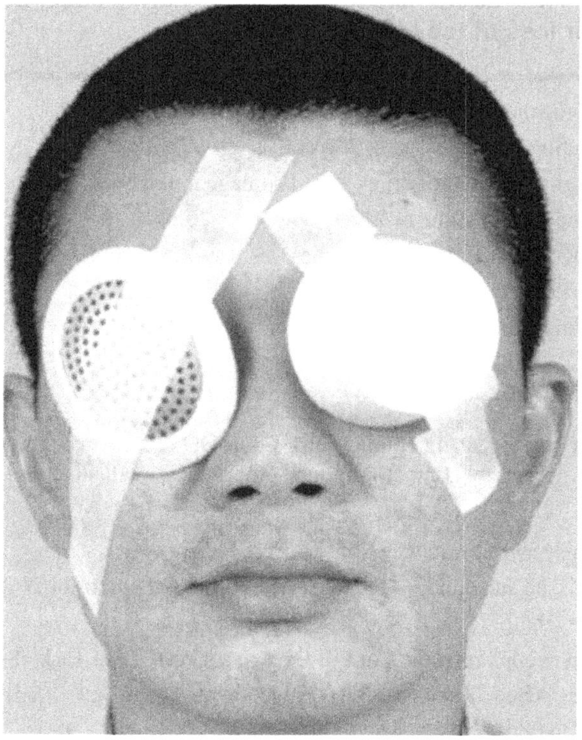

Figure 24-1. Rigid eye-shield or cup properly secured over the injury.

CAUTION

ALWAYS use a rigid eye-shield to provide a barrier to prevent further damage, and NEVER place anything under the rigid eye-shield or directly on the eye.

24-7. Preserve any avulsed (detached) skin or tissue in clean sterile gauze soaked in saline (if available) and transport it with the casualty for possible grafting.

24-8. Cover the uninjured eye with a bandage to decrease movement.

Note. In hazardous conditions (such as combat or unsure footing), leave the good eye uncovered long enough to ensure the casualty's safety.

SEEK EVACUATION AND MEDICAL AID

24-9. While seeking medical or casualty evacuation, do not cause further injury—

- **Limit** movements that could cause further injury to the eye.
- **Do not** administer medication to prevent coughing, sneezing, or vomiting.

24-10. Consider giving the antibiotic tablet provided in the combat pill pack if medical treatment will take more than three hours from the time of injury and if giving the medication to the casualty does not cause nausea.

24-11. Record first aid administered on the DD Form 1380 (provided in the IFAK).

24-12. Evacuate the casualty as follows:

- Transport the casualty on his back, with the head elevated and immobilized.
- Evacuate eyeglasses with the casualty, even if they are broken.

24-13. Do not cause further injury to the eye or casualty while waiting for evacuation. Provide assurance to the casualty and stay with the casualty until relieved by medical personnel or competent authority.

This page intentionally left blank.

★Chapter 25

Initiate First Aid for Foreign Bodies on the Eye (081-833-0039) With IFAK Eye-Shield

SURVEY

25-1. Survey the situation, if the injury is from chemical exposure, immediately wash the eye (see Task 081-833-0044). Otherwise, DO NOT put anything on the eye ITSELF, especially if you think the eye is cut. Examine the eyes as follows:

- Look at the eyes—are the pupils equal and round?
- Look for bleeding or foreign bodies in the eye.

> **WARNING**
>
> **DO NOT put pressure on the eye or remove anything from the eye surface. This could cause additional harm, such as loss of an eye.**

- Foreign bodies in the eye are treated by appropriate medical personnel, or by the casualty if it can easily be removed (for example a surface nonembedded material such as an eyelash or speck of dirt).

SHIELD

25-2. Use the rigid eye-shield provided in the IFAK, the joint first aid kit, or anything that provides a hard cover over the eye, such as—

- Eye protective gear—ballistic glasses or goggles.
- The bottom of a disposable cup, for example one made of extruded polystyrene (foam), plastic, or paper.

Note. This helps prevent any undue pressure or further damage to the eye. DO NOT put any pressure on the eye.

- Secure the rigid eye-shield by applying tape from the cheek to the forehead (see Figure 24-1 on page 24-2). If no tape is available, use gauze, cloth dressing, shoelace or string to secure in place.

> **CAUTION**
>
> ALWAYS use a rigid eye-shield to provide a barrier to prevent further damage, and NEVER place anything under the rigid eye-shield or directly on the eye.

> **CAUTION**
>
> Removing foreign bodies from the eye is NOT a first aid procedure. If tactically possible and terrain permits, place a rigid eye-shield on both eyes and seek medical treatment.

Note. In hazardous conditions (such as combat or unsure footing), leave the good eye uncovered long enough to ensure the casualty's safety.

FOREIGN BODY STUCK OR IMPALED IN THE EYE

CAUTION

DO NOT attempt to remove a foreign object stuck to or sticking into the eyeball. A medical officer (physician) must remove such objects.

25-3. Apply dry sterile dressings to build around and support the object. This will help prevent further contamination and minimize movement of the object. Perform the following:

- Cover the injured eye with a paper cup or cardboard cone.
- Cover the uninjured eye with a dry dressing or eye patch.
- Reassure the casualty by explaining why both eyes are being covered.

Note. The eyes move together. If the casualty uses (moves) the uninjured eye, the injured eye will move as well. Covering both eyes will keep them still and will prevent undue movement on the injured side.

SEEK EVACUATION AND MEDICAL AID

25-4. Seek further medical aid immediately.

25-5. Obtain details about the injury—

- Source and type of foreign bodies if known.
- Whether the foreign bodies were windblown or by what type of high-velocity mechanism.
- Time of onset and length of discomfort.
- Any previous injuries to the eye.

25-6. Do not cause additional injury to the eye—

- Do not probe for foreign bodies.
- Do not put pressure on the eyeball.
- Do not remove the impaled object.
- **Limit** movements that could cause further eye injury.
- **Do not** administer medication to prevent coughing, sneezing, or vomiting.

25-7. Consider giving the antibiotic tablet provided in the combat pill pack if medical treatment will take more than three hours from the time of injury and if giving the medication to the casualty does not cause nausea.

25-8. Record the first aid administered and other information as required on the DD Form 1380 (provided in the IFAK).

25-9. Do not cause further injury to the eye or casualty while waiting for evacuation. Provide assurance to the casualty and stay with the casualty until relieved by medical personnel or competent authority.

★Chapter 26

Initiate First Aid for Extrusions of the Eye (081-833-0042) With IFAK Eye-Shield

SURVEY

26-1. Survey the situation and remove or avoid hazards.

26-2. Remove the casualty's headgear, if necessary.

26-3. Position the casualty as follows:

- Conscious—seated.
- Unconscious—lying on his back with head slightly elevated.
- If conscious, reassure and inform the casualty of the first aid steps that you are providing.

> **WARNING**
>
> **DO NOT put pressure on the eye or remove anything from the eye surface. This could cause additional harm, such as loss of eyesight or loss of the eye.**

26-4. Examine the eyes for the following:

- Objects protruding from the eye or eyes.
- Swelling or lacerations of the eyes.
- Bloodshot appearance of the eyes.
- Bleeding—
  - Surrounding the eye.
  - From inside the eyeball.
  - Coming from the eyeball.
- Contact lenses. Ask the casualty if he is wearing contact lenses, however, do not force the eyelids open.
- Extrusion (the eye is protruding from the socket).

> **CAUTION**
>
> DO NOT attempt to reposition the eyeball or replace it in the eye socket.

SHIELD

26-5. Provide appropriate first aid for the injury as follows:

- Position the casualty face up.
- Cut a hole in several layers of dressing material, and then moisten it. Use sterile water if available, or use the cleanest water available, preferably potable.
- Gently place the dressing so the injured eyeball protrudes through the hole, with minimal contact. Use just as much gentle movement of the dressing as necessary, to surround and protect the eyeball. The dressing should be built up higher than the eyeball.

Note. If available, place a paper cup or cone-shaped piece of cardboard over the eye. This material should not touch the eye. Do not apply pressure to the injury site. Apply roller gauze to hold the cup in place.

- Cover the uninjured eye to prevent sympathetic eye movement.
- The provided IFAK rigid eye-shield will not be deep enough to properly protect the eye extrusion injury. However, the rigid eye-shield may be used to cover the uninjured eye.

Note. In hazardous conditions (such as combat or unsure footing), leave the good eye uncovered long enough to ensure the casualty's safety.

SEEK EVACUATION AND MEDICAL AID

26-6. Call for medical aid immediately and arrange for medical evacuation as soon as possible.

26-7. While calling for medical or casualty evacuation—

- **Limit** movements that could cause further eye injury.
- **Do not** administer medication to prevent coughing, sneezing, or vomiting.
- Consider giving the antibiotic tablet provided in the combat pill pack if medical treatment will take more than three hours from the time of injury and if giving the medication to the casualty does not cause nausea.

26-8. Record the first aid provided on the DD Form 1380 (provided in the IFAK).

26-8. Evacuate the casualty as follows:

- Transport the casualty on his back, with the head elevated and immobilized.
- Evacuate eyeglasses with the casualty, even if they are broken.

26-9. Do not cause further injury to the eye or casualty while waiting for evacuation. Provide assurance to the casualty and stay with the casualty until relieved by medical personnel or competent authority.

★Chapter 27

Initiate First Aid for Chemical Burns of the Eye (081-833-0044) With IFAK Eye-Shield

SURVEY

27-1. Reassure the casualty and quickly survey the situation.

27-2. Quickly identify the substance that the casualty was exposed to such as—

Note. Do not delay first aid to perform this step. Time is critical and the eyes must be irrigated as soon as possible.

- Alkali—the most dangerous of all substances due to the penetrating factor. Common substances that contain the hydroxides of ammonia, lye, potassium, magnesium, and lime—
  - Fertilizers.
  - Cleaning products, drain cleaners, and oven cleaners.
  - Plaster and cement.
- Acid—usually less severe than alkali burns. Common acids contain sulfuric acid, hydrochloric acid, nitric acid, acetic acid, chromic acid, and hydrofluoric acid—
  - Glass polish, vinegar, and nail polish remover.
  - Automobile battery acid.
- Irritants—substances that have a neutral pH tend to cause more discomfort to the eye than actual damage—
  - Most household detergents.
  - Pepper spray.

WARNING

DO NOT put pressure on the eye or remove anything from the eye surface. This could cause additional harm, such as loss of eyesight or loss of the eye.

27-3. Check for the following signs and symptoms:

- Irritation.
- Pain and redness.
- Watering and tearing.
- Possible erosion of the corneal surface.
- Inability to keep the eye open.
- Swelling of the eyelid.
- Blurred vision.

SHIELD

27-4. Initiate first aid for the chemical burn as follows:

- IMMEDIATELY flood the eye with water.
- Keep irrigating the eye with running water from a faucet, low pressure hose, bottle, cup, or intravenous setup (if available). Hold the irrigating tip 1 to 1½ inch away from the casualty's eye or eyes, direct the irrigating solution gently from the inner eye (nearest the nose) to the outer eye away (towards the ear) from the casualty's unaffected eye.
- Start the transport and continue washing out the eye or eyes for at least 20 minutes or until the casualty's arrival at the medical treatment facility.
- Dry the area around the eye or eyes by gently patting with gauze sponges or other appropriate clean material. Do not touch the casualty's eye.
- Cover the injured eye or eyes with the rigid eye-shield provided in the IFAK, the joint first aid kit, or an appropriate device that provides a hard cover over the eye such as—
  - Eye protective gear—ballistic glasses or goggles.
  - The bottom of a disposable cup, for example one made of extruded polystyrene (foam), plastic, or paper.

Note. This helps prevent any undue pressure or further damage to the eye.

- Secure the rigid eye-shield by applying tape from the cheek to the forehead (see Figure 24-1 on page 24-2). If no tape is available, use gauze, cloth dressing, shoelace or string to secure in place.

Note. In hostile environment (such as combat or unsure footing), the eyes may have to remain uncovered so the casualty can see to get away from danger.

Note. Burned eyelids swell to protect the underlying eyes. The eyes should be protected with the rigid eye-shield to prevent further injury.

CAUTION

ALWAYS use a rigid eye-shield to provide a barrier to prevent further damage, and NEVER place anything under the shield or directly on the eye.

SEEK EVACUATION AND MEDICAL AID

27-6. Seek medical evacuation for casualty.

27-7, Do not cause further injury to the eye—

- **Limit** movement that could cause further eye injury.
- **Do not** administer medication to prevent coughing, sneezing, or vomiting.

27-8. Consider giving the antibiotic tablet provided in the combat pill pack if medical treatment will take more than three hours from time of injury and if giving the medication to the casualty does not cause nausea.

27-9. Record the first aid given on the DD Form 1380 (provided in the IFAK).

27-10. Evacuate the casualty without causing further harm.

Appendix A

Improved First Aid Kit

A-1. Improved first aid kit (Figure A-1) contents includes—

- Modular Lightweight Load-carrying Equipment (MOLLE) II, utility pouch.
- Tourniquet, combat application.
- Bandage kit, elastic.
- Bandage gauze, 4½″ 100's package.
- Adhesive tape surgical, 2″ x 6' roll.
- Airway, nasopharyngeal.
- Glove, patient exam, 100's package.
- Dressing, combat gauze.
- Insert, (folding panels with cord).

A-2. See the United States Army Medical Materiel Agency Web site for more information on the IFAK and IFAK II.

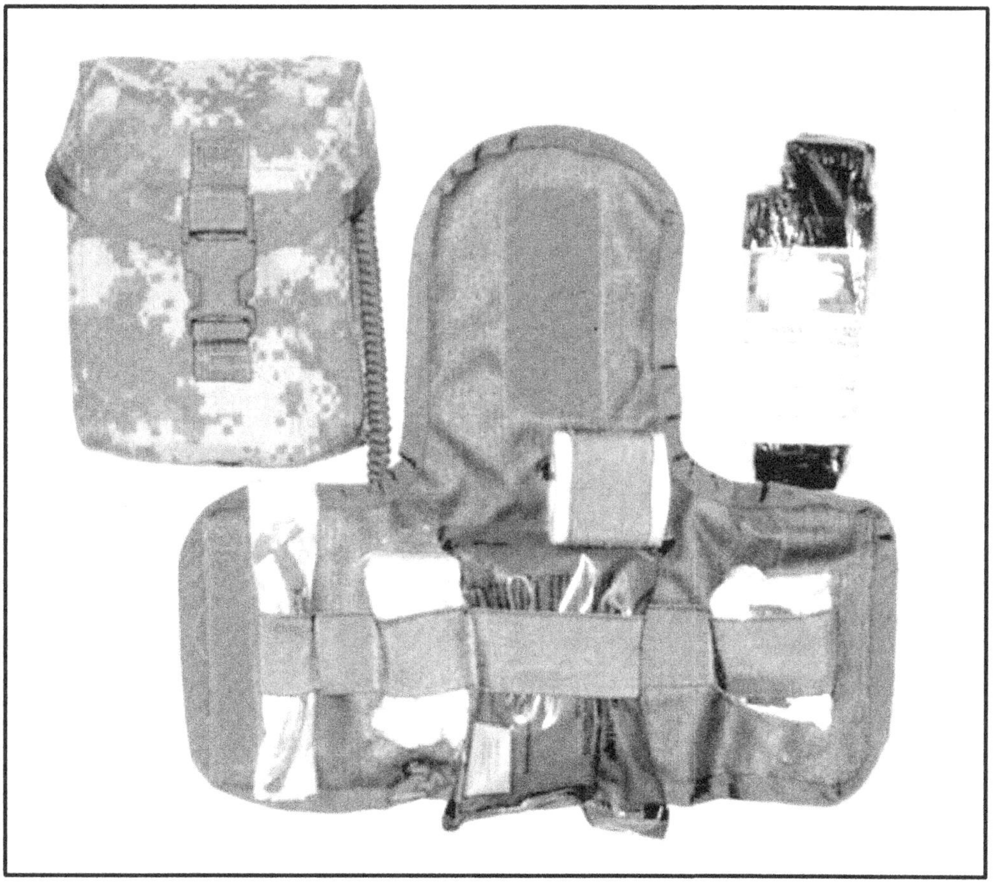

Figure A-1. Improved first aid kit

A-4. The IFAK II (Figure A-2) adds—

- 1 new custom pouch.
- Second tourniquet, combat application.
- 1 marker.
- 1 eye shield.
- 1 commercial chest seal.
- 1 strap cutter.
- 1 TCCC Card (DD Form 1380).
- Combat gauze is issued by the unit.

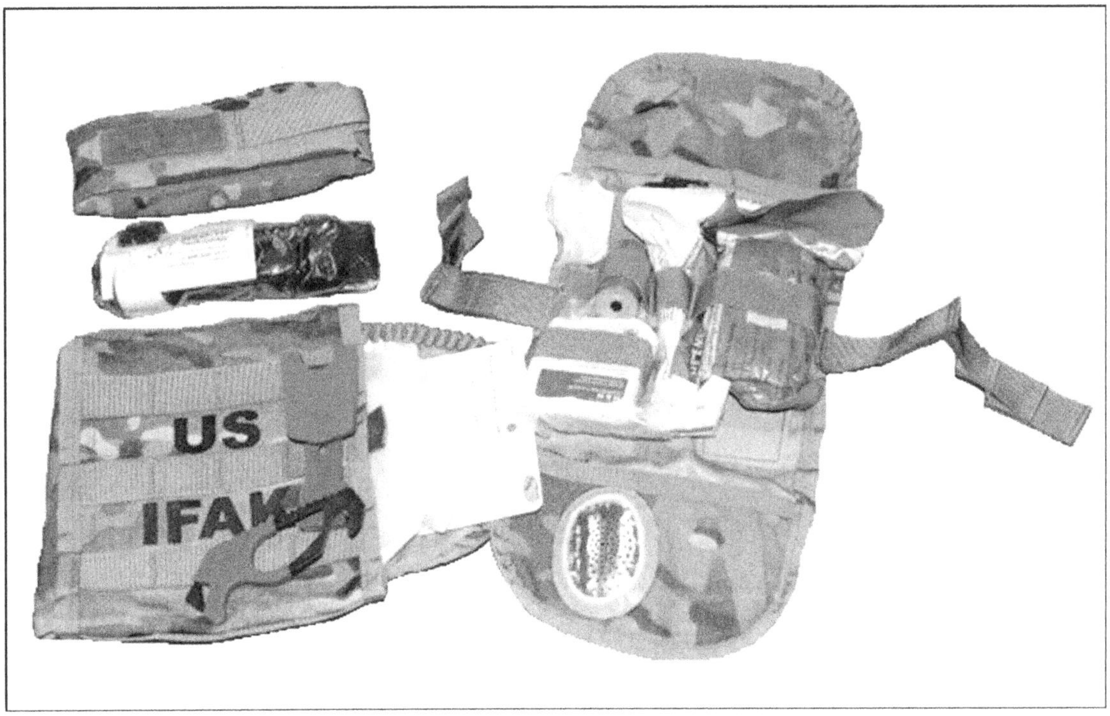

Figure A-2. Improved first aid kit II

Glossary

This glossary lists acronyms and terms with Army or joint definitions. This publication is not the proponent for any terms.

SECTION I – ACRONYMS AND ABBREVIATIONS

AMedP	Allied medical publication
ATNAA	antidote treatment nerve agent autoinjector
ATP	Army techniques publication
CANA	convulsant antidoate for nerve agent
CASEVAC	casualty evacuation
DA	Department of the Army
DD	Department of Defense
F	Fahrenheit
FM	field manual
CPR	cardiopulmonary resuscitation
DOD	Department of Defense
IFAK	improved first aid kit
JSLIST	Joint Service Lightweight Integrated Suit Technology
MOS	military occupational specialty
NATO	North Atlantic Treaty Organization
NPA	Nasopharyngeal airway
STANAG	standardization agreement
STP	Soldier training publication
TC	training circular
TC3	tactical combat casualty care
TCCC	tactical combat casualty care card

This page intentionally left blank.

References

REQUIRED PUBLICATIONS

These documents must be available to the intended users of this publication.

These publications are available online at http://www.apd.army.mil. Accessed on 28 October 2015.

ADRP 1-02, *Terms and Military Symbols*, 7 December 2015.

STP 8-68W13-SM-TG, *Soldier's Manual and Trainer's Guide, MOS 68W Health Care Specialist, Skill Levels 1, 2, and 3*, 3 May 2013.

STP 21-1-SMCT, *Soldier's Manual of Common Tasks, Warrior Skills, Level I*, 10 August 2015.

These publications are available online at http://www.dtic.mil/doctrine. Accessed on 28 October 2015.

JP 1-02, *Department of Defense Dictionary of Military and Associated Terms*, 8 November 2010.

RELATED PUBLICATIONS

These documents contain relevant supplemental information.

NATO STANDARDS AND STANDARDIZATION AGREEMENTS

These publications are available online at http://nso.nato.int/nso/. Accessed on 28 October 2015.

Standard, AMedP-8.12, *Military Acute Trauma Care Training, Edition A, Version 1*, July 2015.

STANAG 2122, *Requirement for Training in First Aid, Emergency Care in Combat Situations and Basic Hygiene for all Military Personnel*, Edition 3, 11 November 2010.

STANAG 2126, *First-Aid Dressings, First Aid Kits and Emergency Medical Care Kits*, Edition 6, 10 December 2009.

STANAG 2358, *First Aid and Hygiene Training in a Chemical, Biological, Radiological, and Nuclear or Toxic Industrial Hazard Environment*, Edition 4, 5 January 2009.

STANAG 2544, *Requirements for Military Acute Trauma Care Training*, Edition 2, 14 July 2015.

ARMY PUBLICATIONS

Most Army doctrinal publications are available online at http://www.apd.army.mil. Accessed on 28 October 2015.

ATP 4-02.2, *Medical Evacuation*, 12 August 2014.

ATP 4-02.3, *Army Health System Support to Maneuver Forces*, 9 June 2014.

ATP 4-25.12, *Unit Field Sanitation Teams*, 30 April 2014.

ATP 4-25.13, *Casualty Evacuation*, 15 February 2013.

ATP 5-19, *Risk Management*, 14 April 2014.

★ ATP 6-22.5, *A Leader's Guide to Soldier Health and Fitness*, 10 February 2016. Accessed on 8 June 2016.

FM 4-02, *Army Health System*, 26 August 2013.

FM 27-10, *The Law of Land Warfare*, 18 July 1956.

TC 4-02.3, *Field Hygiene and Sanitation*, 6 May 2015.

WEB SITES

★ Joint Theater Trauma System Clinical Practice Guideline. http://www.usaisr.amedd.army.mil/cpgs/Initial_Care_of_Ocular_and_Adnexal_Injuries_24Nov2014.pdf Accessed on 8 June 2016.

United States Army Public Health Center. (Heat Illness Prevention)
https://phc.amedd.army.mil/TOPICS/DISCOND/HIPSS/Pages/HeatInjuryPrevention.aspx
(Cold Weather Casualties and Injuries)
http://phc.amedd.army.mil/topics/discond/cip/Pages/ColdCasualtiesInjuries.aspx

United States Army Medical Materiel Agency. http://www.usamma.amedd.army.mil/assets/docs/IFAK.pdf and http://www.army.mil/article/116565

★ Vision Care of Excellence http://vce.health.mil/. (Click on "Service Members and Veterans" tab, go to "Related Contents," select "Eye Injury Response Tips.") Accessed on 8 June 2016.

PRESCRIBED FORMS

None.

REFERENCED FORMS

Unless otherwise indicated, Department of the Army (DA) Forms are available on the Army Publishing Directorate (APD) Web site (www.apd.army.mil). Accessed on 10 November 2015.

DA Form 2028, *Recommended Changes to Publications and Blank Forms.*

Department of Defense (DD) Forms are available on the Office of the Secretary of Defense (OSD) Web site (www.dtic.mil/whs/directives/infomgt/forms/formsprogram.htm). Accessed on 10 November 2015.

DD Form 1380, *Tactical Combat Casualty Care (TCCC) Card.*

Index

References are to paragraph numbers except where otherwise specified.

This page intentionally left blank.

TC 4-02.1
21 January 2016

By Order of the Secretary of the Army:

MARK A. MILLEY
General, United States Army
Chief of Staff

GERALD B. O'KEEFE
Administrative Assistant to the
Secretary of the Army
1601105

DISTRIBUTION:

Active Army, Army National Guard, and United States Army Reserve: Distributed in electronic media only (EMO).

PIN: 106005-000

Made in the USA
Monee, IL
08 November 2026

67380772R00066